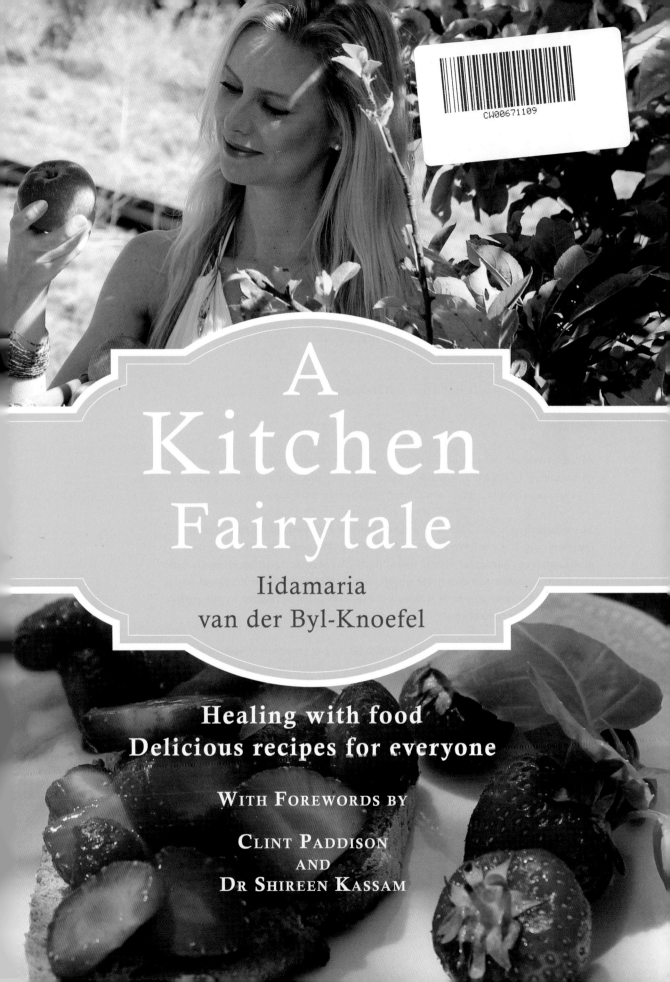

A Kitchen Fairytale

Iidamaria
van der Byl-Knoefel

Healing with food
Delicious recipes for everyone

WITH FOREWORDS BY

CLINT PADDISON
AND
DR SHIREEN KASSAM

First published in 2018 by Hammersmith Health Books –
an imprint of Hammersmith Books Limited
4/4A Bloomsbury Square, London WC1A 2RP, UK
www.hammersmithbooks.co.uk

© 2018, Iida van der Byl-Knoefel (text and photographs)

Reprinted 2018

All rights reserved. No part of this publication may be reproduced, stored in a retrieval system, or transmitted in any form or by any means, electronic, mechanical, photocopying, recording, or otherwise without the prior written permission of the publishers.

The information in this book is of a general nature and is meant for educational purposes only. It is not intended as medical advice. The contents may not be used to treat, or diagnose, any particular disease or any particular person. Applying elements from this publication does not constitute a professional relationship or professional advice or services. No endorsement or warranty is explicitly given or implied by any entity connected to this content.

As always, if you are have pre-existing health issues and especially if you are taking any medications, you are advised first to consult your health practitioner before making any changes to your lifestyle and diet.

British Library Cataloguing in Publication Data: a CIP record
of this book is available from the British Library.

Print ISBN: 978-1-78161-134-0
Ebook ISBN: 978-1-78161-135-7

Editor: Georgina Bentliff
Cover design: Madeline Meckiffe
Text designed and typeset by: Madeline Meckiffe, Julie Bennett and Iida van der Byl-Knoefel
Production: Helen Whitehorn of Path Projects Ltd
Printed in Poland on behalf of One World Books Ltd

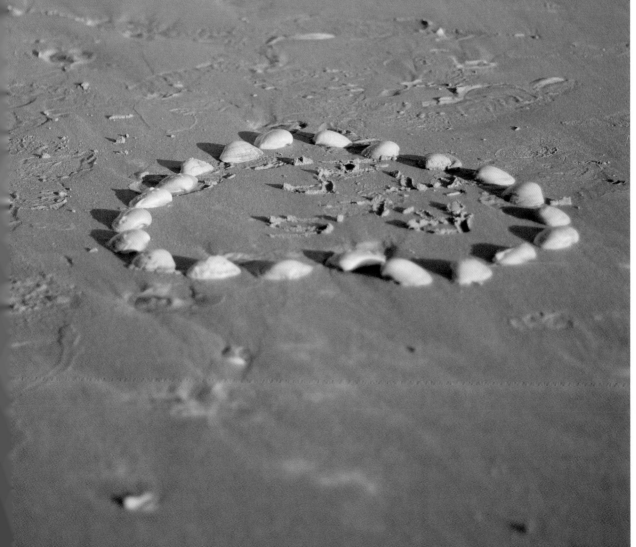

Dedication

To Fred
For being the best person in the world,
for walking next to me throughout this journey
and for contributing to this book by always
spotting any lack of crunchiness in a recipe

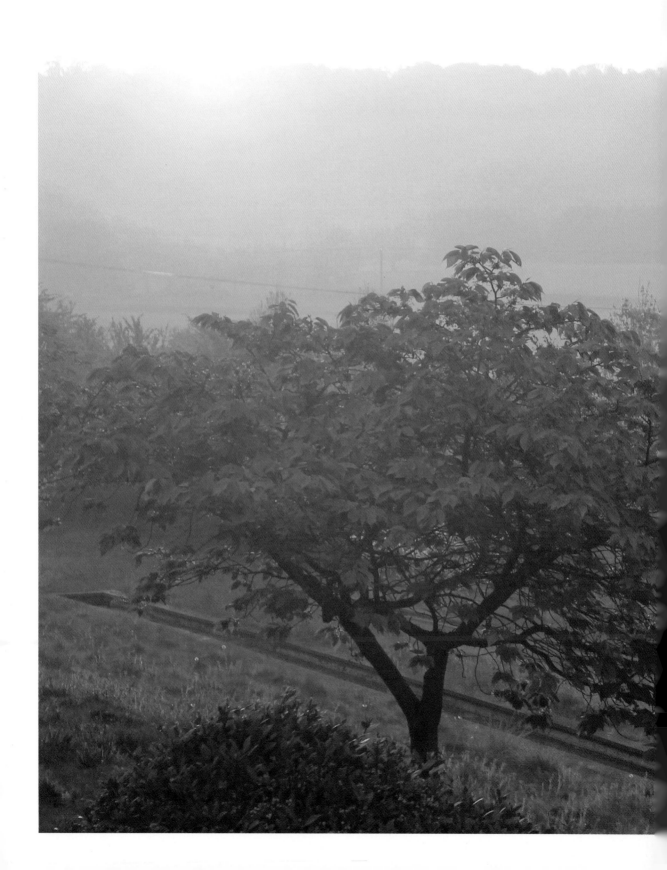

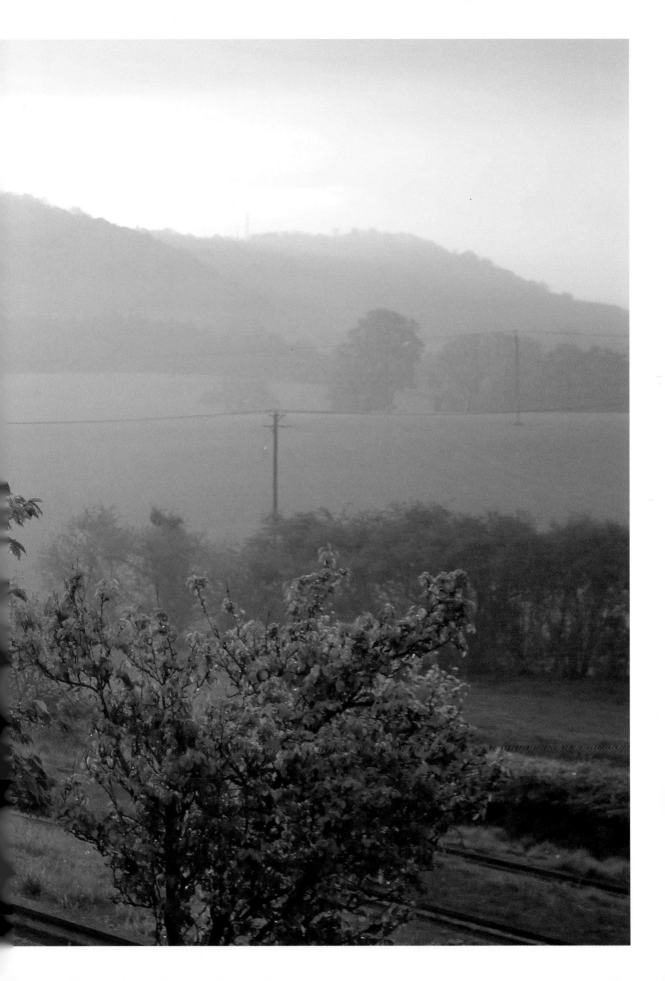

Contents

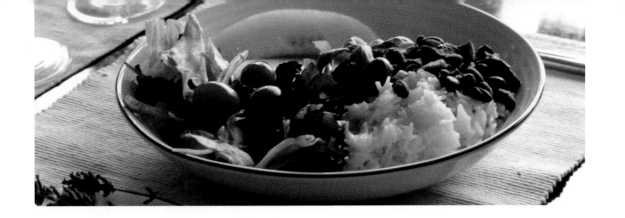

———✦———

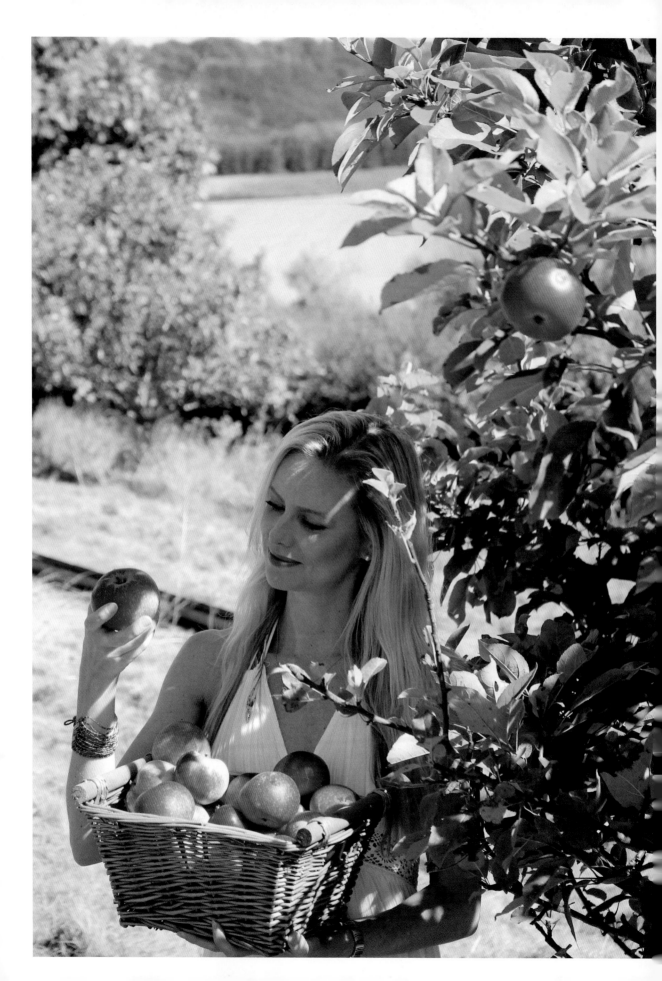

Forewords

Iida is a breath of fresh air to the plant-based community. She is driven by a sincere passion to help others after recovering from a very serious autoimmune condition and adopting ground-breaking measures to treat it naturally.

Iida and I first met on my Paddison Podcast, where she shared her incredible health transformation. What struck me about Iida was that she had grand plans for the future. She spoke with excitement about 'what's next' and provided her view of a happier, healthier world through a plant-based diet. The episode with Iida was far reaching, and the combination of her kind nature, health recovery, and sound knowledge of autoimmune fundamentals inspired thousands of people worldwide.

Since then she has garnered a large loyal audience, who admire her work equally as health advocate, plant-based chef, and photographer with a girl-next-door like-ability. So it was only a matter of time until she pulled together the best of her cooking and photography work and presented it for the benefit of others on a grander scale.

It's an honour to introduce Iida's *A Kitchen Fairytale* to the world.

It's bright. It's light. It's fresh, and it's brimming with potential for what can be in the future.

Not just for the person Iida will become, as a highly popular voice of clarity in the clouded space of nutrition, but also for the broader human race. For *A Kitchen Fairytale* presents wholesome, delicious, beautiful recipes that come wrapped up in a big, warm bundle of hope. Hope for what can be achieved on an individual level when we follow the right plan and make healing a must – alongside the hope for what might be achieved as a civilisation if we were to follow her eating style. *A Kitchen Fairytale* recipes will make the human race healthier, reduce our collective carbon footprint dramatically, and correct the erroneous view that animals are a necessary food.

Enjoy *A Kitchen Fairytale* and feel proud, joyful and righteous that you're consuming plant-based foods. Because it is the way of the future, and with Iida's labour of love it's now become tastier than ever.

Clint Paddison, founder of *The Paddison Program for Rheumatoid Arthritis*

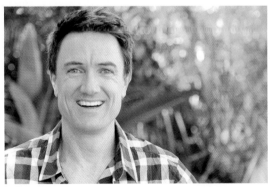

I am honoured to be able to write this dedication in support of this wonderful book. Iida and I met through our shared passion for promoting plant-based nutrition for optimal health and wellbeing. Iida has healed her own body through plant-based nutrition and is now committed to helping others heal too.

The urgency of the plant-based message cannot be overstated. We are in the midst of a full-blown epidemic of diet-related chronic disease. The human race is fatter and sicker than ever before. The most common causes of death and disease, including cardiovascular disease, cancer, diabetes and hypertension, are directly related to the food we eat. Studies suggest that up to 70% of chronic disease could be prevented by making lifestyle changes, with diet changes being of greatest importance. So where have we gone wrong? Since the end of the second World War, the diet of well-resourced Western countries has become increasingly defined by high amounts of animal-derived and processed foods. This has been made possible by the advent of industrialised agriculture and fast-food outlets. Our demand for these foods is also contributing to the destruction of our planet and its natural resources. The shift from a predominantly plant-based, low-calorie, nutrient-dense diet to one that is calorie dense, yet nutrient deficient is fuelling the rise in chronic disease. As under-resourced countries become more affluent, they are adopting the food habits now prevalent in the West, with devastating, yet predictable, consequences. Medical advances, remarkable though they are, rely on pills and procedures to help control the symptoms of disease, yet most conventional medical treatments fail to address the root cause – our diet.

Iida's journey back to health using a dietary approach is remarkable and inspiring. Yet it should not come as a surprise. We have known for decades that many common diseases can be prevented and reversed by adopting a predominantly whole-food plant-based diet, low in added fat, salt and sugar. In addition to arthritis, scientific studies have reported reversal of diseases such as severe coronary artery disease, diabetes, early stage cancer, inflammatory bowel disease and other autoimmune diseases through the adoption of a diet made up of vegetables, whole grains, legumes and fruits. Some of the longest lived, healthiest populations in the world are eating a predominantly unprocessed diet of whole plant foods rich in fibre and other plant nutrients and low in animal fat and protein.

In this book, Iida shares her knowledge and expertise with recipes that will help you and your family enjoy delicious, health-promoting food. Share this book with everyone that you can, because Iida's story should not be a secret. We all have the power to heal our body through food and in doing so we will begin to heal our planet.

Dr Shireen Kassam
Consultant Haematologist, London, UK

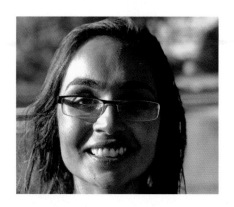

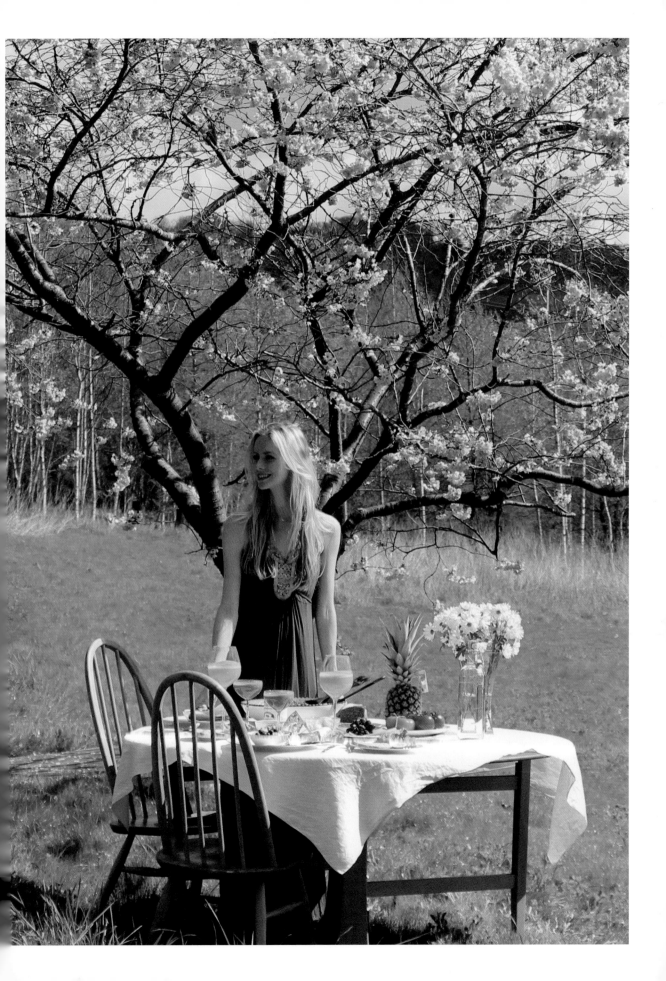

Welcome

Welcome to a world of delicious and healing plant-based foods. I have been creating these recipes while healing my body from inflammatory arthritis, very similar to rheumatoid arthritis; a chronic disease I was told, until I turned it around with a change in diet.

All the recipes in this book are humble and nourishing, as well as delicious and mostly very easy to make. For me, and for so many others, moving onto a plant-based diet has turned out to be a tremendously satisfying experience and I can now see how people have thrived on eating like this for thousands of years. There is nothing new about going plant-based; rather, it is a move back to a humble diet that has worked for us humans throughout history, without all the artificial nonsense that is put into our foods today.

So if you are new to plant-based cooking, I am absolutely delighted to see you here, and I hope that you will enjoy widening your senses and learning all about this wonderful way of cooking.

If you are already plant-based, I am equally pleased to see you here and I hope that this book will give you some further inspiration in the kitchen.

Iida

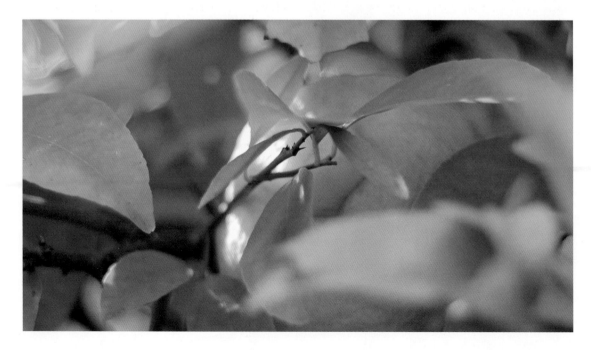

My story

I used to think that I had a healthy diet; I would have a good breakfast of salmon, spinach and eggs, or rye bread with a slice of cheese/ham/turkey and veggies, or yoghurt and granola. I would avoid ready-made meals and processed foods as much as I could, and choose full-fat dairy products, because who knows what goes into the low fat ones? I wouldn't deprive myself of 'treats', so every now and then I would have a burger with fries, some ice cream or pizza, and Sunday roasts were always a great end to the week.

I also ventured into the world of low-carbohydrate, high-fat and protein, because everyone is always talking about how carbohydrates make you put on weight and leave you bloated, causing high blood sugar spikes that then send you crashing down, longing for something sweet. Lean protein in the shape of white meat and fish would surely be the way to build a strong, healthy body, right?

Well, that didn't work so well for me, and at the age of 32 I developed a form of inflammatory arthritis, similar to rheumatoid arthritis (RA); in simple terms a state where my joints were being attacked by my own immune system.

From July 2014 until August 2015 I suffered from this vicious disease which made my left knee so swollen that I had to walk down the stairs with my left foot first, as my left knee wouldn't bend far enough to take a normal step. Some days I could hardly walk the four minutes to the grocery shop and I had to decline invitations to concerts and other events with my friends, because I knew that I wouldn't be able to stand up for more than a few minutes before my knee began to swell. I nevertheless had the same energy as before, and wanted to do everything that I had been used to, so having my body shut down on me like that was a horrendous experience.

Doctors, osteopaths, homeopaths, acupuncturists and physiotherapists were all unable to help relieve my pain and a year after the onset of the symptoms, in the summer of 2015, I started taking the medication sulfasalazine, as prescribed by the rheumatologist. This was probably the most awful experience to date; I felt like I had metallic poison going through my veins and it gave me a terrible, unnatural headache, unlike anything that I had experienced before. After two weeks I ended up in the emergency room having had an allergic reaction to the medication. I stopped taking it immediately and that is when I decided to get well on my own.

I embarked on my own intensive research to see if the condition could be healed naturally and I noticed that whenever others indicated that they had recovered from rheumatoid arthritis, there would be a mention of dietary change. I began by excluding dairy, gluten and sugar, and greatly increased the anti-inflammatory foods in my diet. Not only did the latter result in a decrease in pain and inflammation, but it also made my cooking extremely tasty – and this involved simple ingredients like garlic, ginger and turmeric!

Around the same time I also discovered yoga and so clearly remember how some very simple exercises took away the pain within 10 minutes (see the yoga stretch that helps my knees on page 16). I started doing yoga every morning and evening at home – 10 minutes to an hour each session. The swelling in the knee went down and the pain around my body started disappearing; I could feel the difference immediately.

Less than a month after implementing these changes I went to see my rheumatologist, who told me that my blood test results showed that I was back to normal. Hearing her tell me this was just beyond amazing, as it showed that the natural approach had worked, where the drugs had not. I told her my story, expecting her to say that the results had nothing to do with the change in diet but on the contrary, and to my surprise, she told me to continue and also asked if she could pass on my recommendations to her other patients who were asking for a natural way of beating the disease, to which I happily agreed.

However, I still knew that I hadn't been able to get to the bottom of the disease because though a lot of the symptoms had gone away with the initial food elimination, persistent inflammation that wasn't attributable to any one food still lingered.

I also wanted to remove the fear of being stricken by this disease again. After further online research, I found the Paddison Program for Rheumatoid Arthritis (PP) where Clint Paddison addresses the underlying cause of the condition before presenting steps to help heal the body from the inside and give it the chance to reverse various forms of inflammatory arthritis. What Clint Paddison brought to light, and which I hadn't discovered during my own research, was that the severity of my own immune system attacking my joints was being increased by fat and undigested proteins in my diet. The remaining inflammation was therefore resolved by going through the elimination process of the PP, followed by long periods of eating gut-healing foods and doing certain types of exercise. As a result, since October 2015 I have been on a no-oil, whole-foods plant-based diet, where fruits, vegetables, whole grains and legumes take centre stage. I have excluded all meat, fish, egg and dairy products, as well as vegetable oils, because extracted oils, being pure fat, interfere with the digestive system. After several months on the PP, I was able to reintroduce foods with higher fat content, like nuts, olives, coconut and avocados, that had previously caused swelling in various joints; as a result, the recipes in this book reflect this progression.

The PP was crucial to my healing process and as an added bonus it steered me in the direction of a plant-based lifestyle. I do, however, recall how hard it was to start cooking in such a different way; this book is my means of sharing some of the delicious recipes that allowed my body to continue to heal after the initial phases of the PP. Following on from the foundation principles of the PP, these recipes do not

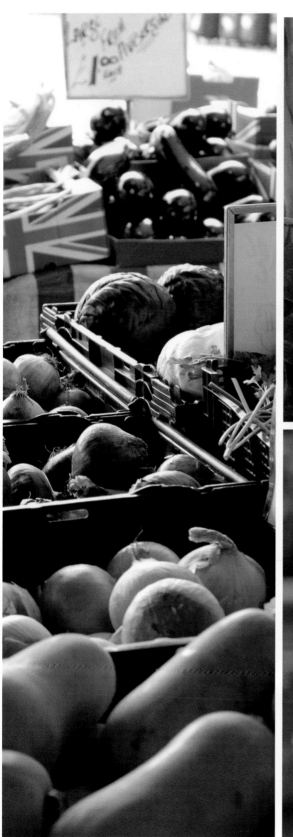
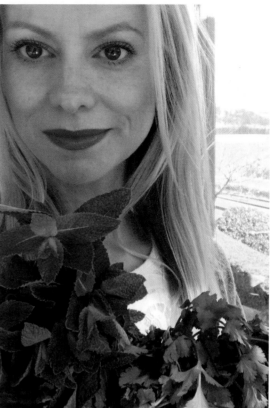
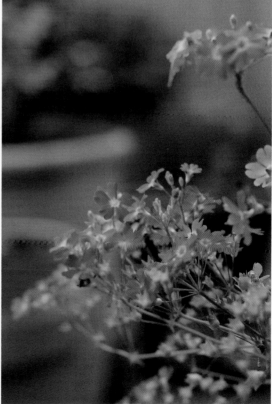

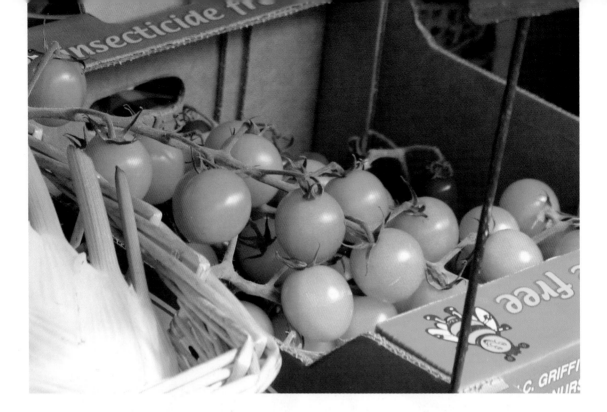

contain any animal-derived products or oils that may aggravate the healing process.

This diet works like a dream; the symptoms of arthritis have disappeared and my test results are back to normal, which is something that the doctors very rarely, if ever, see. The inexplicable stomach pains and irritable bowel syndrome which I used to experience are also gone. I never get cravings for sweet 'treats' because my body is so satisfied with all the goodness that it derives from whole foods, and I have considerable amounts of energy.

Yoga and exercise

I started using the cross trainer at the gym in February 2016 and my knee responded well very quickly and grew increasingly strong while the pain and swelling subsided further. I would hop on it 3-4 times a week for 30 minutes; I initially started on the lowest resistance and within a couple of months I had worked my way up to the highest resistance. This was followed up with some lighter weight training, a lot of stretching and yoga.

My favourite yoga stretch for the knees

Lie flat on your back on the floor, breathe in deeply and bring your knees up towards your chest. At the same time, lift your head and upper back from the floor, and reach for the bottom of your feet with both hands. Hold your feet and your breath for five seconds, then let go, lean back and lower your legs and head back onto the floor slowly while you breathe out. Repeat five times. You can alternate by lifting up one foot at a time.

This was the exercise which made the most positive impact on my knee at the very beginning of my journey. It also helped me discover yoga, as it immediately took away the pain in my knee and left it pain free for several hours. Initially I couldn't get my knees anywhere near my chest, as one in particular was so swollen, but after about a month or two I was able to rest my knees on my chest – great proof that the exercise was helping.

I still do this move about five times a week.

Where I am today

I haven't taken any medication since those two weeks in August 2015. Overall, the inflammation which caused the arthritis is gone and my test results remain normal, including iron and calcium levels. Healing the body naturally is a slower process than we are used to with modern medication, where pain and symptoms are quickly masked. With inflammatory arthritis, the workings of my gut were essentially harmed from the food that I used to eat, so I am still in the process of healing my gut, slowly reintroducing foods and observing how my system reacts to them. Eating something too high in protein or fat results in a slight swelling in a finger or knee, but this recedes after a few hours.

I expect to eat like this for a while longer, gradually introducing new foods and enjoying the ones which I can tolerate.

Once my gut is completely healed, I feel sure that I shall remain a happy plant-based eater for the rest of my life, given how great it makes me feel and knowing the positive effect which it will have on my future well-being. I have learned to listen to my body in a way which I had never expected, and if something feels wrong, I try to establish why that is, instead of rushing for painkillers or other drugs which we use so liberally these days.

We sometimes have to take medicine and are fortunate to live in times where science in that field is so advanced. However, I find that we often rush to treat the symptoms instead of investigating the underlying causes of so many of our modern-day diseases, and this therefore often keeps people on medication for the rest of their lives, even though there is an alternative solution close at hand. The established medical profession acknowledges the connection between diet and certain diseases, and it is also therefore logical that we should seek solutions to various other conditions in a plant-based diet.

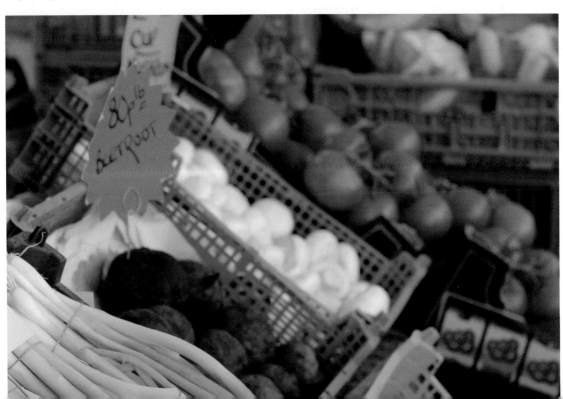

A plant-based diet and disease today

The body is such a remarkable instrument, always working to heal itself. Just think about when you accidentally cut your finger and how quickly it heals – we don't even question whether it will heal or not, we just know it does. The same process happens on the inside, where constant healing is taking place; in my case, given the right conditions, my dysfunctional digestive system was able to heal, leading to the end of arthritis.

We hear about miracle cures for everything these days so I know how daunting it can be to read about yet another way of fixing the problem. For me, however, learning about a plant-based, whole-food diet just made such sense and observing how quickly my body reacted to it finally convinced me.

I like to think about it like this: we humans are part of nature and have been living ever so close to it for millennia. These days, however, with our modern cities with their amazing, advanced technology, it is small wonder how easy it is to forget how complex nature is, including the foods which are part of it. The nutrients in whole foods are so beautifully balanced that, when we consume them in their natural state, we obtain all the nutrients which our bodies require to function properly.

Today however, so much is readily available in a pre-packaged form that we have moved away from the nutrition which we evolved to eat. During the course of evolution our ancestors most likely wouldn't have started their days with large cups of caffeinated drinks filled with sugar and dairy, and they probably wouldn't recognise half the ways that meat is processed and presented as foods these days.

We also tend to eat like kings and queens three times a day, so no wonder our bodies are taking the strain and manifesting discontent through different diseases. The most distressing aspect is seeing these illnesses starting to affect younger and younger people.

While we continue to eat our super-delicious processed, ready-made foods we also experience all these health problems, and turn our attention to miracle cures, be they single nutrients in the shape of supplements to prevent specific diseases, or pills and drugs which suppress the symptoms, or diets promising a quick fix.

At the moment, some of the most popular diets are the high-protein, high-fat ones – I should know, because I was cutting down on carbohydrates like bread and pasta, and

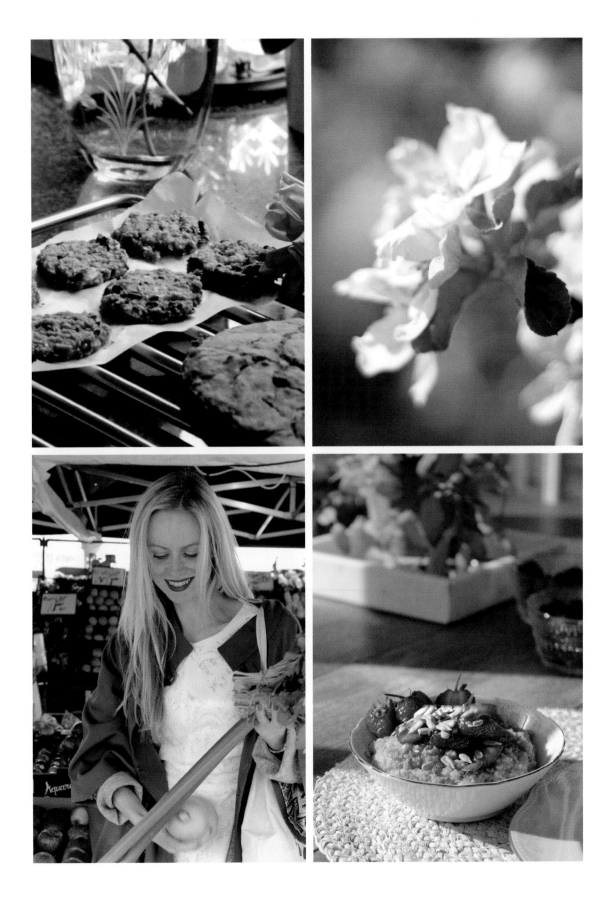

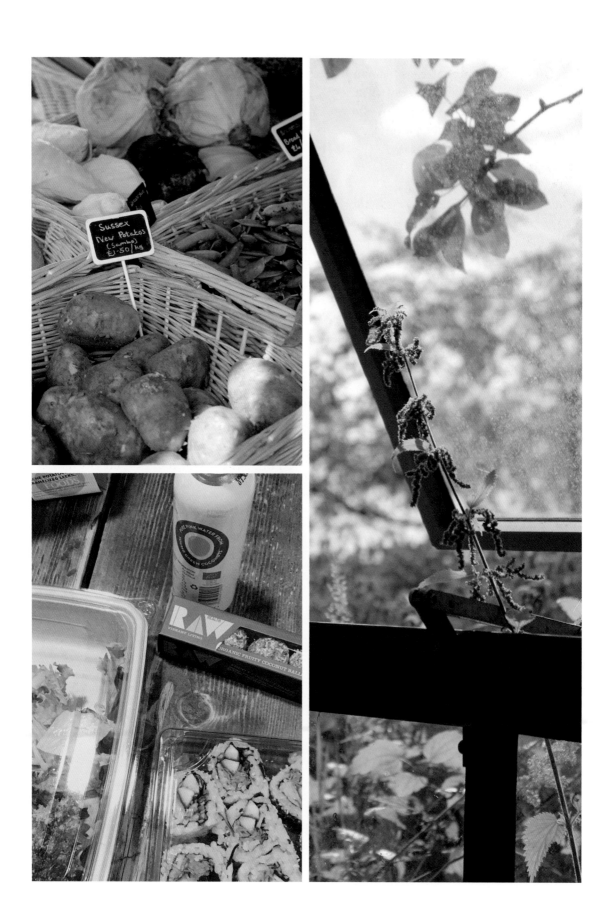

increasing the amount of eggs, fish and white meat before I became so very sick. Increasing evidence, however, now shows that it is the vast amount of animal protein in our diet that is the direct link to many of the health disorders we are facing.[1]

The day I was prescribed medication for arthritis was the day on which it occurred to me that the emphasis on palliative care rather than addressing the underlying root causes was a strategic error. I eventually realised that all along I had been aggravating my system with the very foods that I thought were keeping me healthy, and how grateful I was to learn that I could stop the vicious circle by swapping all the animal-based foods for a rainbow of grains, vegetables and fruits. I am nevertheless grateful that I had a quick stint on medication, because during the first few weeks of changing my diet, which can be tough with only very humble foods on the menu that allow the gut to heal, I was able to think back to how awful the medication had made me feel, and suddenly that spoon of buckwheat tasted mighty delicious. Now, with the profound adaptation of my taste buds, buckwheat tastes amazing as it is.

More and more doctors around the world are moving into lifestyle medicine and guiding their patients through a transition to a plant-based diet to prevent, halt and even reverse conditions like diabetes and heart disease, which have been considered chronic. These patients also routinely report improvements in other conditions, like osteoporosis, high cholesterol, high blood pressure, cancer, multiple sclerosis, autoimmune diseases (been there!), headaches, acne, asthma, allergies, colds and inflammatory bowel disease, to name but a few.[2]

Dr Colin T Campbell goes into great scientific detail about the link between animal protein and disease in the book *The China Study.* In *Forks Over Knives,* Alona Pulde, MD, and Matthew Lederman, MD, further explore why we are so unwell despite all the advanced science and modern technology now available, and Dr McDougall's website is loaded with free information on how various health conditions are improved as well as cured and reversed with a plant-based diet, in addition to welcoming people on-site with more hands-on guidance.

Just to add another angle to the high-protein diet debate, we all know by now that the amount of meat which we currently consume in the Western diet has a profoundly negative impact on the environment. This should make any one of us stop to reflect on whether that steak on our plate is worth it. I for one wouldn't want my children, nieces or nephews to look at me one day and ask why we didn't do anything, even though we knew that our actions were directly harming their future.

What can I expect from a plant-based diet?

This cookbook is a collection of all the recipes created while healing my gut. Each chapter includes foods that I was able to tolerate early on as well as more advanced recipes for wwhen the gut is able to tolerate a wider range.'

The recipes that I have found to be kindest to the system have been labelled with a *'Humble and healing'* sign and those are the recipes to which I return whenever I want to reset my body – for example, after having done a lot of travelling and fallen out of my regular routines.

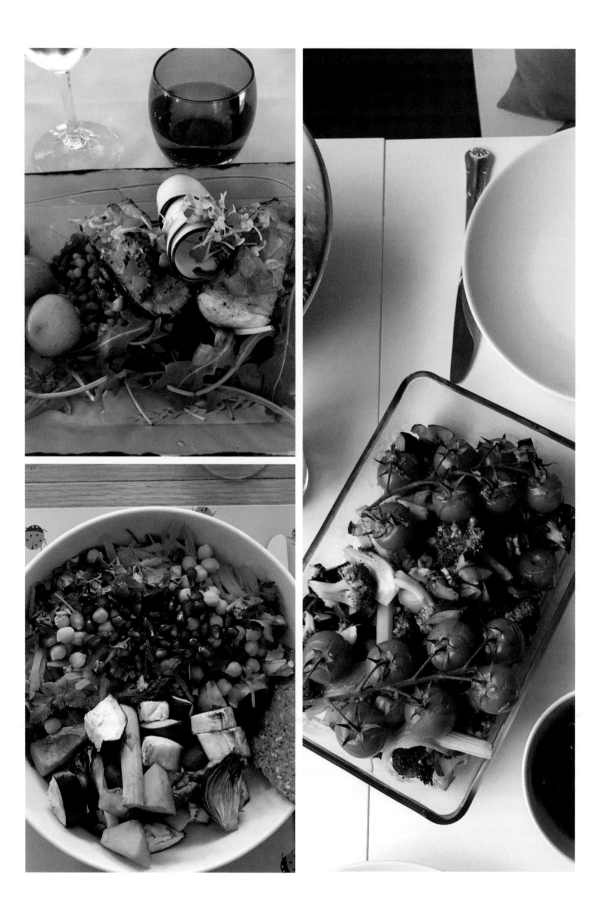

One day of eating these basic foods is usually enough to stop any inflammation and get back into balance, and I can then continue where I left off. During all this time, the symptoms have kept diminishing steadily, so I know that eventually falling out of routines won't have any effect on my health. For now, I am still careful with the foods I know I am still reacting to slightly – mainly lentils – but when I do have them I make sure to add a huge bunch of baby spinach or kale to help break them down in my gut.

If you are on the Paddison Program, the best approach is to follow the first four phases of the Program exactly as directed – after that, all the recipes in this book are an expansion of everything which you can eat beyond that point.

When it comes to healing the gut, our tolerances are individual, so the important thing is to pay attention to how the foods make *you* feel and not to rush into trying too many new foods in one go. If there is anything in these recipes which you cannot yet have, simply exclude that ingredient or replace it with foods that you can tolerate; patience is key and eventually you will be able to have all of these whole foods again. For example, I wasn't able to eat bell peppers for years as they used to give me severe stomach aches, but now that I have given my gut the chance to heal, these vegetables are back on the menu again, to my great surprise and delight.

I know very well how intimidating it sounds to stop having meat and dairy – so what is there left to eat? Well, first and most importantly, when eating like this you will not go hungry or feel unsatisfied and your system will get all the vitamins, minerals, fats, proteins and carbohydrates that you need. Within a few days you may notice that small issues which have bothered you health-wise are easing up, and this might be just the push that you need to keep going. Do have a look through this book and maybe challenge yourself to follow a plant-based diet for a month to see how you get on. A month out of your whole life is really no big deal; you can definitely do it! Resetting your body like this and giving it a rest from processing all that heavy food will always be a good thing, so don't be afraid to give it a go.

In my experience, the biggest difference when going plant-based was that I had been used to seeing my meals based around meat or fish, with maybe some potatoes or rice and veggies on the side. Suddenly, centre stage of my plate was taken up by potatoes, sweet potatoes, rice, pasta, grains or bread – with lots of beautiful vegetables, beans, lentils and nuts as accompaniment. I also learned to incorporate a great deal of fermented foods, as they contain probiotics which will help improve the immune system and the digestive function. My favourite ones are brown rice miso, kimchi and sauerkraut and I do also take probiotic capsules every day to further help my gut to heal.

After going plant-based I very quickly decided that I didn't want to miss out on my favourite foods, so I made a conscious effort to create plant-based versions of dishes that we all love, like lasagne, burgers, chillies, stir-fries and pasta with various sauces, and you will find them all in this book.

It has been a fascinating and unexpected journey to relearn everything that I thought I knew about nutrition and health. I know that it is confusing to get your head around this new way of thinking after a lifetime of learning that dairy gives strong bones, and meat brings us iron, but seeing such significant results within a short space is what convinced me. Moving onto a plant-based diet wasn't the easiest thing for me and it took a good three months to stop craving meat and dairy; only after that did I no longer get food envy when others were having "normal" food. While writing this I am a year in and I have no desire to go back to my old ways; my body tells me how happy it is on a whole-foods diet by working the way it was designed to.

One of my favourite parts of going plant-based began a few weeks into changing my ways; the flavours in food became more intense and complex, and today, when I eat something as simple as an organic orange, it is the most wonderful taste experience. I have found that extracting more intense enjoyment out of the simplest things gives an extra level of happiness to life.

Protein, iron, calcium and vitamins

The most common question I am asked is, 'Where do you get your protein from?' closely followed by, 'How about iron and calcium?' so I thought I should shed some light on this. On a plant-based diet where we consume unprocessed foods that are as close to their natural state as possible, the body derives all the protein that it needs through complex metabolic systems.[3] (By 'unprocessed' foods I mean, for example, boiled potatoes, sliced avocado and shredded carrots – nothing has been extracted or added.)

Protein

Protein is an important nutrient required for the building, maintenance and repair of tissues in the body. Protein consists of 20 different amino acids, 12 of which can be synthesised naturally by our bodies. The remaining eight are called 'essential' amino acids because they need to be obtained from foods – we can't make them. Plants contain an abundance of these eight essential amino acids and they are only found in meat and dairy products because these animals have eaten plants. To put it into perspective; the largest animals obtain all the protein that they require from plants; so the human need for protein is therefore easily met by eating a variety of whole grains, beans, vegetables and fruits.[4]

'… it's not a mystery that we've evolved over millions of years without ever aiming for a "source" of this [protein] or any other nutrient. Yet the mistaken notion that we need to go out of our way to consume certain individual nutrients is pervasive, and protein is the nutrient most commonly identified as one you must target to ensure you get enough. But we're not interested in trying to achieve arbitrary targets; we're interested in achieving good health. And the best way to achieve good health is by targeting whole plant foods, not numbers of grams of protein.'
The Forks Over Knives Plan[5]

It seems that to some extent the confusion today lies in the amount of protein that we should consume. The recommended daily allowance (RDA) of protein is far less than many of us think; on average it is 0.8 grams per kilogram of body weight.[6]

For a person weighing 55 kg, the RDA is 44 grams of protein – an amount easily met on a plant-based diet as long as calorie intake is sufficient.

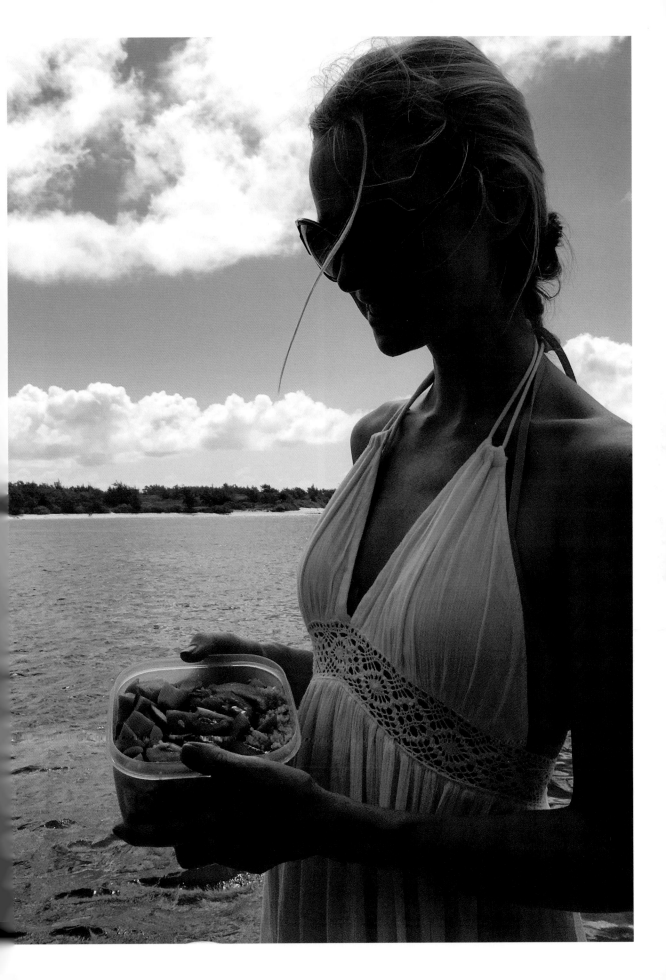

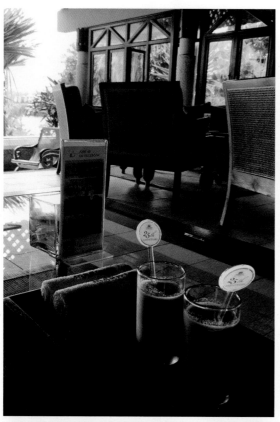
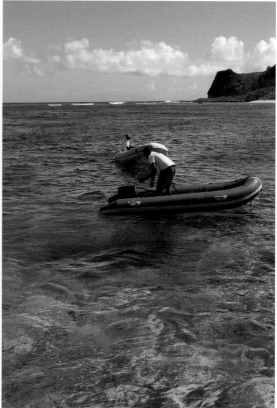
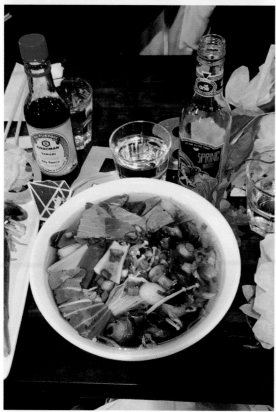
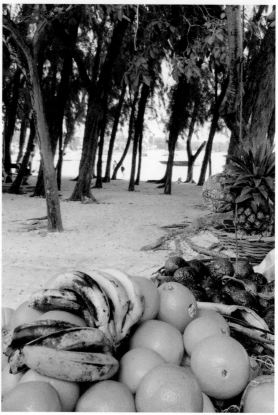

Calcium

I was taught at an early stage that I needed to drink milk and eat cheese so that my body could build strong bones, so despite starting out life as a lactose-intolerant baby, I eventually ended up consuming quantities of dairy products like the people around me. I believe in my case, dairy consumption was a significant contributing factor to getting so very sick, and within two weeks of stopping my dairy intake in August 2015, my test results from the rheumatologist returned to normal. So where should we derive our calcium if not from dairy products?

Calcium is a mineral found in the soil, which plants absorb through their roots before incorporating it into their various tissues; roots, stems, leaves, flowers, and fruits[7]. Once I started on the Paddison Program and researched a plant-based diet further, it was revealing to learn that the best sources of calcium are in fact plants like bok choy, broccoli, cabbage and kale, and that calcium in plants is more easily absorbed by the body than that in cow's milk. I was also surprised to learn that the parts of the world with the lowest dairy consumption, Africa and Asia, also exhibit the lowest rates of osteoporosis. When we consume animal protein, the acid load in the body increases, and the body will try to neutralise the acid with a base (alkali) – calcium being an effective one. Calcium is drawn from the bones, weakening them and increasing the risk of fractures.[8] A plant-based diet doesn't create this kind of acidic environment, consequently decreasing the risk of fractures.

Iron

We have also learned that we get iron from meat; however, we get sufficient iron from a plant-based diet, without all the downsides of consuming high amounts of animal protein. Good sources of plant-based iron include beans and lentils, broccoli, leafy green vegetables, quinoa, brown rice and oats. The absorption of iron is increased when the meal contains a good source of vitamin C, also contained in vegetables like broccoli and bok choi, which renders them excellent sources of iron.[9]

Vitamin B12 and vitamin D

There are 13 vitamins which our bodies cannot synthesise and therefore need to be obtained through our diet. Of these vitamins, two are not produced by most plants: vitamin B12 and vitamin D. The sun is the best source of vitamin D; we can make this vitamin in our skin by spending 15-30 minutes in the sun every few days without any sun block;[10] we just have to make sure not to overexpose ourselves to UV radiation, which increases the risk of other health problems.

The plant-based doctors do encourage us to monitor our B12 levels on a regular basis when on a plant-based diet. At one point in history we obtained vitamin B12 from the soil on vegetables which hadn't been properly cleaned, but these days we wash everything so thoroughly that this is no longer a source for us.[11]

Dr McDougall and Dr T Colin Campbell both recommend very small doses of B12 supplements.

How to succeed in sticking to a plant-based lifestyle

A great motivator for me was to think where I should like to see myself in a year's time: do I want to make the effort of staying on a limited diet for a while now or would I prefer to find myself a year from now, in the same pain and agony, still munching away on the 'ordinary' foods which caused the problem in the first place? That was an easy decision to take and I was positively surprised to find how satisfying this so-called 'limited' diet was.

The world is still coming to grips with a plant-based diet as a lifestyle, so it can be a challenge to find the foods that you are looking for, mainly when eating out. However, the demand is growing and as more people ask for plant-based food, more plant-based cafés and food shops, and options at regular restaurants, are appearing. I know nevertheless how hard it is to stick to a certain diet – what do you eat when you are at a restaurant or at someone's house?

Well, for me it has been easy during this time because I absolutely couldn't eat anything outside my remit, or my body would go into pain immediately. So I have learned just to call the restaurant before my visit and tell them that I am on a medical diet and cannot have meat, dairy or oils. They have been extremely helpful and prepared some delicious meals for me, which have further inspired my own cooking.

When going for a meal at a friend's house I have often just brought my own food, and then spent a very interesting lunch answering questions, most of the time awakening an interest among the other guests about the direct effect of food on our health and well-being. Whenever my friends have offered to cook for me it has always resulted in the most wonderful dishes that all the other guests have helped devour – you can see some of the pictures featured in this book. This has inspired many of my friends to start cooking more plant-based dishes and I love hearing their stories about how they, as a result, have started feeling better in various ways.

If you feel that you miss having some creamy porridge or milk with your hot drink, there are always ways of getting around it. My favourite plant-based milk to start out with was oat milk, because I was able to have oats quite early on. After about nine months on the Paddison Program, I was able to tolerate nuts and at that point nut milks became a delicious addition. If you can make your own nut milk, I would recommend that you do so, as it is even better than the shop-bought alternatives, but we don't always have the time to make our own, so do find your favourite brands, check the ingredients and go from there.

For many people, cheese is the hardest thing to cut down on or stop having altogether and I was delighted when my cravings disappeared after a few months. This was probably helped by discovering the effect on my system when I ate it. However, a creamy and cheesy pasta sauce has always been a favourite so I created a plant-based recipe which you can find in the pasta-section of the book. It always leaves me replete and has been given the thumbs up by the greatest cheese lover I know.

Gluten

I have been having sourdough spelt and rye bread, which both contain gluten, without the healing process being compromised. I also look forward to eventually incorporating whole wheat bread and pasta into my diet, as they are delicious and have great nutritional value.

Wheat in white pasta and bread, however, has been stripped of so much of its nutritional goodness that I believe an intake of these foods is best limited.

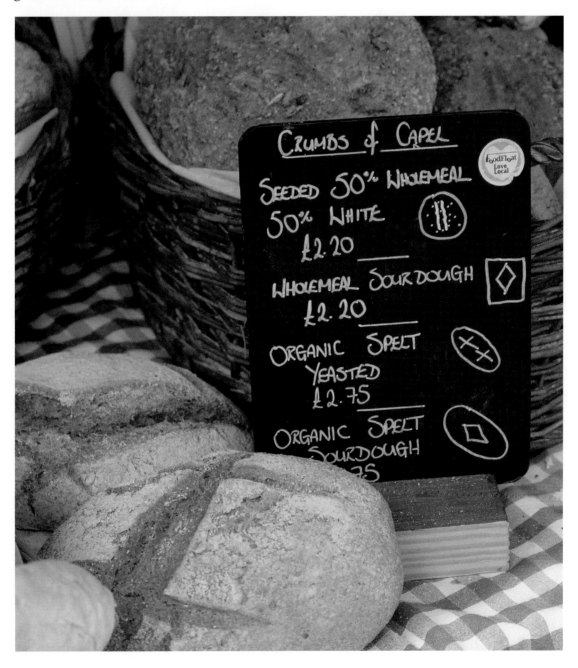

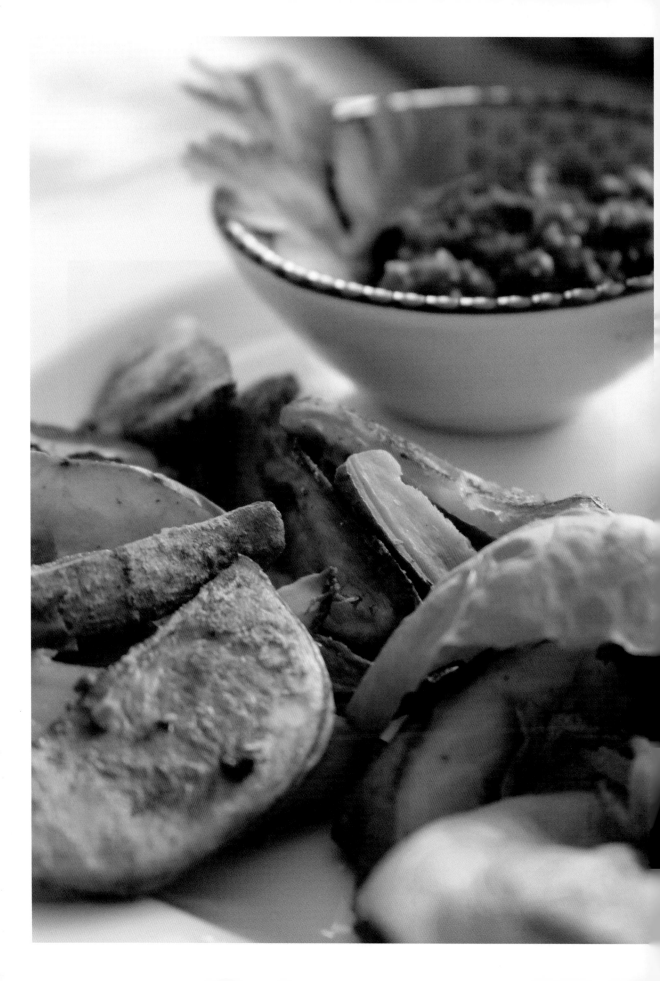

A note about oils and fats

You will soon discover that there are no oils used in any of the recipes in this book; this is following on from the Paddison Program's principles stating that it is essential to exclude all oils from the diet. The fact that I was unable to find any cookbooks that didn't use oils was one of the reasons I decided to write my own. So why are oils so bad for us, when we have been told that many oils are health foods? Let's break it down to the basics to try to make sense of it all.

Whole foods, like coconuts and olives, contain a naturally evolved, balanced mixture of proteins, carbohydrates, fats, vitamins, minerals etc.[12] Oil is made by isolating one single component – the fat – while leaving the fibre, protein and carbohydrates behind, resulting in a highly refined product. Dietary fat causes inflammation in the gut,[13] and the more inflammation in the gut, the more tiny lesions are created in the gut wall, contributing to a worsening of joint inflammation.[14] Many of the plant-based medical doctors advise us to steer clear of oils altogether in order to restore and maintain health and even to reverse various diseases; these include Dr T Colin Campbell, Dr Caldwell Esselstyn and Dr John McDougall. They go into detail about how oils – including olive oil – affect the blood vessels negatively,[15] and are harmful to the innermost lining of the arteries – injury that Dr Esselstyn, for example, refers to as 'the gateway to vascular disease'.[16]

Eating plant foods whole – in their natural state – is the best way to derive all their goodness, including the essential fatty acids (omega-3 and omega-6) that we do need. The no-oil recipes here are humble and kind to the system, allowing healing to take place.

Cooking without oils

So how do you cook without oils? The main use for oils is frying, oven roasting and as an ingredient in salad dressings. These are all easy to get around.

Non-stick pans are the best for frying (I call it 'steam-frying') and ceramic frying pans work especially well when cooking without oils. Just heat a dash of water in the pan, add the vegetables when it starts sizzling and keep adding water during the cooking as needed to prevent anything from sticking to the pan. You can drizzle over some fresh lemon juice and Tamari sauce as well as add chillies and ginger for some lovely flavour. You can also make your own vegetable broth – I have shared my favourite one on page 136. I usually make a huge batch and keep the stock in portion-sized bags or ice cube trays in the freezer, to be taken out and used as necessary.

For roasting in the oven, make sure to choose non-stick oven-proof dishes and always have baking parchment in the house. I also love my re-usable cooking mat as it can be cleaned in a few seconds and stored away until next time. As for oven roasting your foods, just sprinkle some water on top of the veggies before they go in – sometimes you may need to sprinkle some more water on halfway through the cooking time.

You can find a wide range of no-oil salad dressings in the *Side dishes, salad dressings and sauces (page 154)* section of the book.

A note about salt

The recipes will often say to add salt '*to taste*' because that way you can decide how salty you would like the food. I prefer to keep the salt at the table and add it at that point, rather than during the cooking process, as I find this allows you to use less salt with it tasting more. I use Himalayan pink salt because of its nutritional value, containing a wide range of minerals. During my healing process, I also used a herb salt called Herbamare as it is delicious and worked very well for me even during the earlier stages of the Paddison Program.

A note about weights and measures

I have chosen to measure the ingredients in (UK) cups rather than grams because I find it quicker to use a measuring cup rather than weighing all the ingredients. Plant-based cooking also tends to be rather forgiving in terms of amounts and usually the key is getting the proportions rights, rather than the exact measurements.

Breakfasts

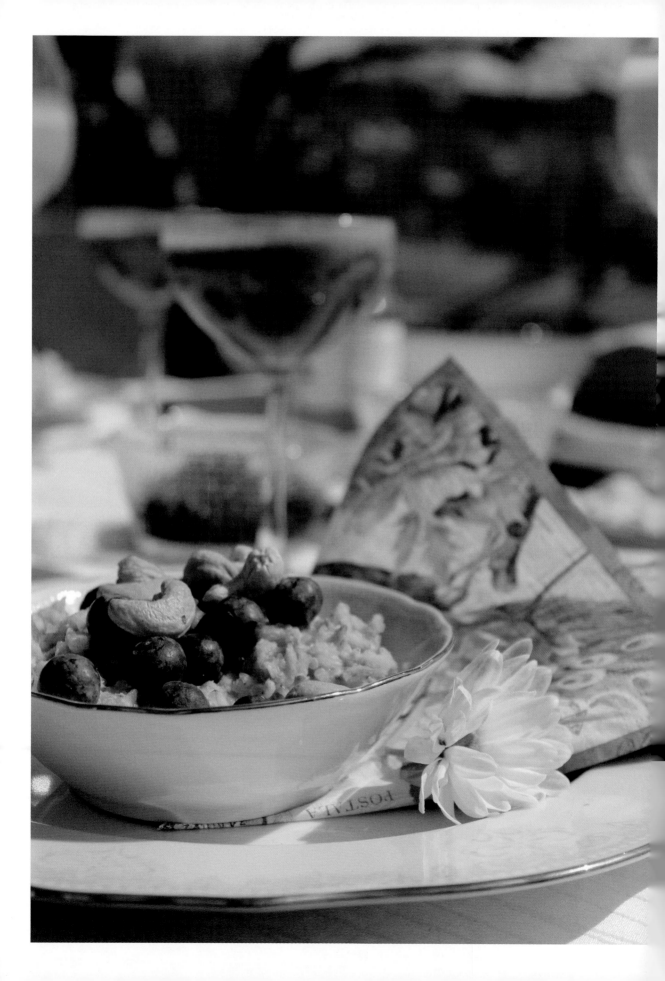

Comforting porridge

Porridge has become my staple breakfast and there are just so many variations that there aren't enough mornings for all this goodness. The portion sizes are rather vague, because on a plant-based diet you just eat until you are full and satisfied. You might in fact find that you eat greater amounts of food than before, but in general the calorie density in whole, plant-based foods is lower, which evens intake out in comparison with non-plant-based food. It is an interesting journey learning to listen to the body's signals and since plant-based whole foods are filled with wonderful nutrients, you will be nourishing your body with every bite.

Porridge base

Quinoa
Buckwheat
Gluten-free rolled oats
Gluten-free jumbo oats
Steel-cut oats

These different grains or pseudo grains can be cooked separately or together in various mixes as they all have different health benefits. I had either quinoa or buckwheat every single day for the longest time and I felt it aid and speed up my healing. I tend to cook a big batch of quinoa and/or buckwheat, as both need to cook for a slightly longer time than regular oats. I then keep them in the fridge and add them to my oats the next morning for a quick and delicious breakfast that keeps me full for hours.

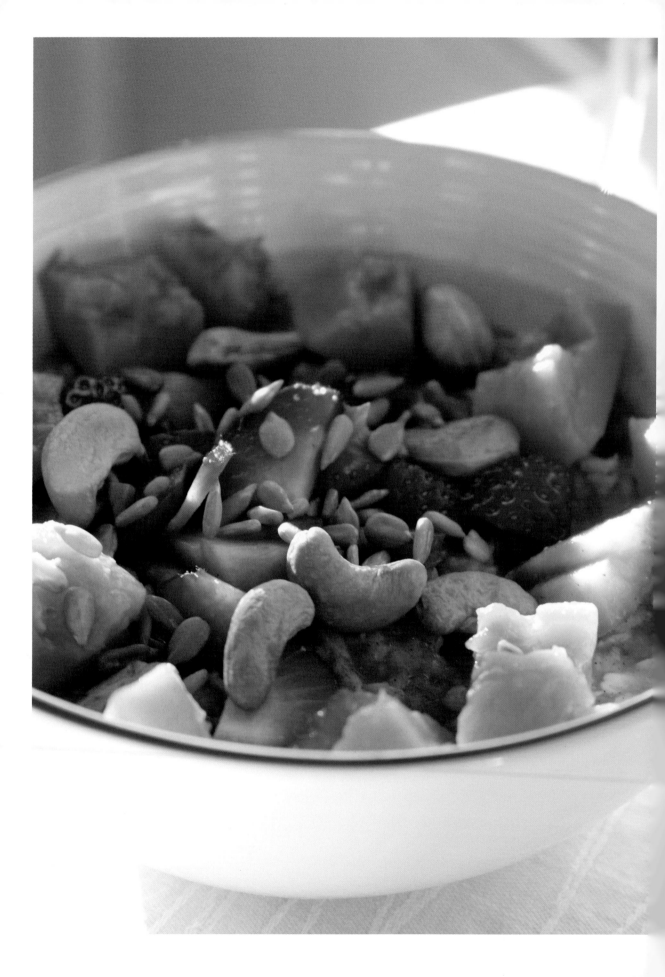

Apple-infused quinoa and buckwheat porridge

This is a really humble recipe which I was able to have quite early on after the initial elimination part of the Paddison Program. Eventually, when I was able to tolerate small quantities of nuts, I would have dry-roasted cashews with it. I also learnt from Clint Paddison that if you are having nuts it is a good idea to have some fresh spinach on the side, as the enzymes this contains will help break down the fats in the nuts, so I always have a green smoothie with my porridge. The quinoa or buckwheat can be exchanged for oats.

SERVES: 2-3

½ cup buckwheat
½ cup quinoa
3-4 cups water
1 grated apple
½ tsp cinnamon

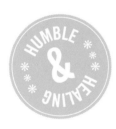

Add the buckwheat, quinoa and water to a pan and bring to the boil.

Cook for approximately 20 minutes or until soft.

Towards the end you can add more boiled water if you wish to have a slightly looser consistency and let the mixture cook for another few minutes.

Stir in the grated apple and cinnamon.

Either serve straight away or let it all warm up on the stove for about 20 seconds before serving.

You can also scatter fruit or berries on top together with dry-roasted cashew nuts.

Enjoy with a green smoothie on the side.

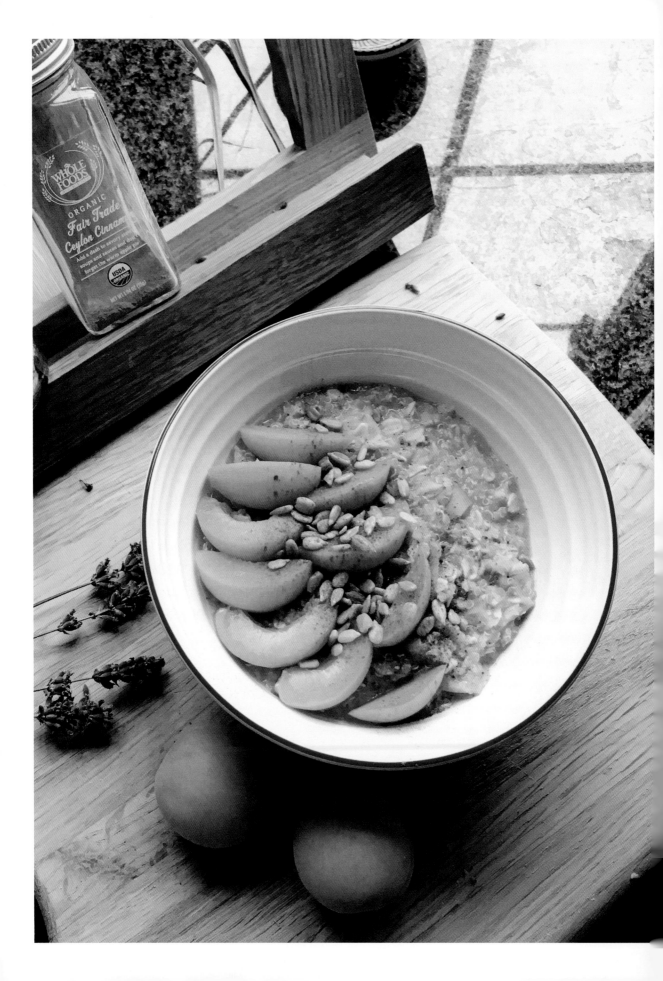

Triple cinnamon porridge

SERVES: 3-4

½ cup buckwheat grouts
½ cup quinoa
4 cups water
½ cup gluten-free rolled oats
1 tsp cinnamon

Add the buckwheat, quinoa and water to a saucepan and bring to the boil. Lower the heat and cook until soft, which takes approximately 20 minutes. Stir every now and then.

With a couple of minutes left of the cooking time, stir in the oats, cinnamon and some more water if the consistency is too thick and simmer until the oats have softened.

Serve with your favourite fruits or berries.

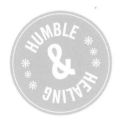

Steel-cut oats and quinoa

Quinoa and steel-cut oats both need to cook for 15-20 minutes and can therefore be cooked together.

SERVES: 2-3

½ cup quinoa
½ cup steel-cut oats
4 cups cold water

Rinse and add the quinoa and oats to a pot with the water, bring to the boil then turn down the heat and simmer until soft, which takes approximately 20 minutes, or less for a chewier consistency.

Serve with your favourite toppings – for example, chopped papaya, mango or sliced banana.

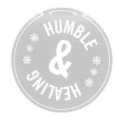

Christmassy rice porridge

In Finland, rice porridge (similar to what is called 'rice pudding' in the UK) is a traditional Christmas Eve breakfast, which is easy to understand, as it makes such a comforting meal on a freezing cold day. Top with either blueberries or the strawberry compote (see page 54).

SERVES: 4

1 cup pudding rice or Arborio
(risotto) rice
½ tsp Himalayan pink salt
1 cinnamon stick
6 cups oat milk
Fresh berries, rinsed

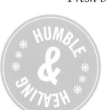

Add the rice, salt, cinnamon stick and oat milk to a pan and bring to the boil.

Turn the heat right down to low and cook for 45 minutes to one hour, stirring occasionally, until the rice is done.

Serve with cinnamon and fresh berries.

Bilberries (like blueberries but smaller) are a perfect topping here. If you don't have fresh ones, buy some frozen ones and either have them as they are or heat them in a pan with a dash of water; just don't allow them to start boiling. Pour over your porridge and enjoy.

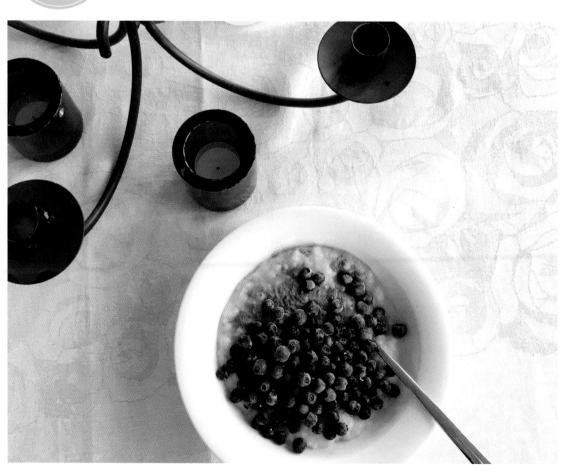

Blueberry, cinnamon and vanilla overnight oats

SERVES: 1

1 medium-sized banana
½ cup oats
¾ cup oat milk
¼ tsp cinnamon
¼ tsp vanilla powder
A handful of blueberries

Mash up the banana in a bowl.

Pour in the rest of the ingredients and stir well.

Cover and place in the fridge overnight.

In the morning, stir through and enjoy with a green smoothie on the side.

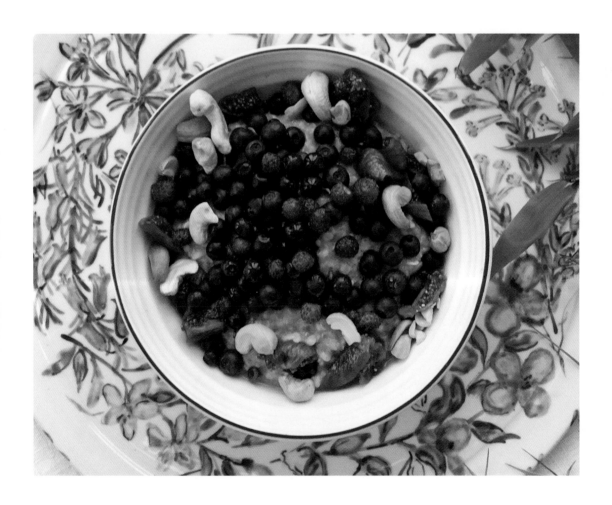

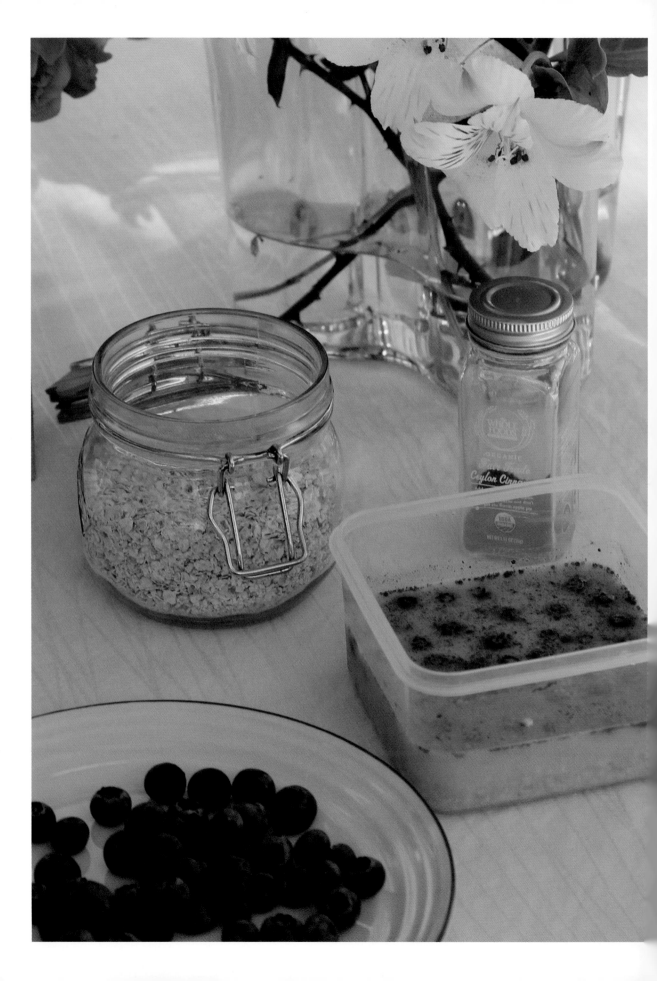

Quinoa, orange and vanilla overnight oats

SERVES: 2

1 orange, peeled
½ cup filtered water
½ cup rolled oats
½ cup quinoa, cooked
1 tsp vanilla powder

In a blender, whizz the peeled orange and the water.

Pour this orange juice into your food container.

Mix in the oats, the cooked quinoa, the vanilla powder and stir until smooth.

Close the lid and place in the fridge over night.

Serve the next morning with, for example: berries / grated apple / sliced banana / chopped papaya / dry-roasted nuts / soaked almonds.

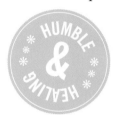

Raspberry overnight oats

SERVES: 1

½ cup gluten-free oats
1 ½ cup oat milk
A large handful of raspberries, rinsed
½ cup quinoa and/or buckwheat, cooked

Place the oats in a food container, pour over the oat milk, add the raspberries and stir well.

Close the lid and place in the fridge over night.

In the morning, mix in your cooked quinoa and/or buckwheat.

Serve with sliced banana, or if it is a cold, wintry day you can warm it all up on the hob on a low heat with a dash of additional oat milk.

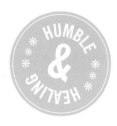

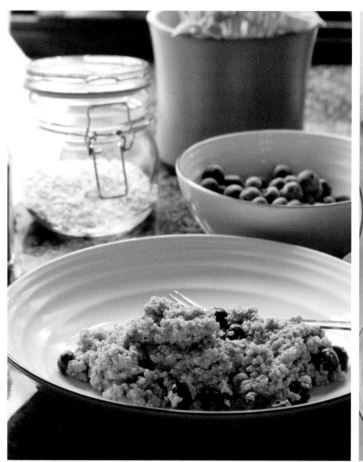

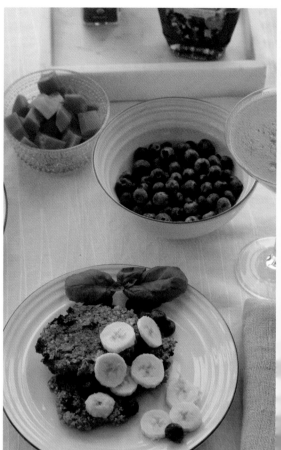

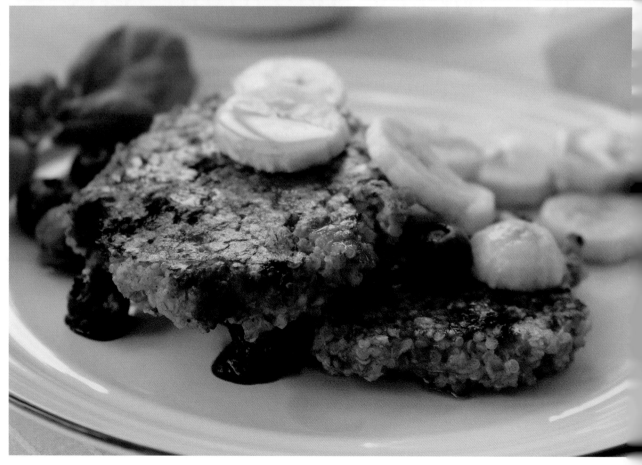

Pancakes

Healing buckwheat pancakes

SERVES: 2

*½ cup quinoa or
buckwheat, cooked
1 cup gluten-free oats
½ - 1 cup water
1 banana
1 tsp cinnamon
A sprinkling of Himalayan
pink salt
Blueberries or raspberries
– optional*

Choice of toppings:
*Chopped pineapple
and fresh basil
Maple syrup
and sliced banana
Your favourite
fruit or berries*

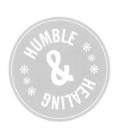

Mix the quinoa or the buckwheat in a bowl with the gluten-free oats and keep adding the water until you have a thick paste or batter.

Mash up the banana and stir into the batter.

At this point you can fold in the berries if you wish to make berry pancakes. You can also just sprinkle the berries on top at the end.

Preheat a pan on the hob (ceramic pans are amazing for cooking without oils as nothing sticks) and sprinkle with some water. Keep on a low heat.

Spoon approximately 2 tbsp of the batter into the pan to form a round pancake.

Cook on a low heat until the pancake starts firming up.

Once firm, bring the heat up to give the pancake some colour, before you carefully flip it over.

Cook on the other side on medium heat until the pancake is firm and cooked through.

As always, enjoy with a green smoothie on the side.

Sunshiny pancakes

I love pancakes and a lot of experimenting and testing resulted in this rustic, delicious recipe with a true pancake-y consistency.

SERVES: 2

2 medium-sized very ripe bananas
1 cup oats
1 cup plant-based milk (I prefer almond or oat milk)
2 tbsp spelt flour
1 tsp bicarbonate of soda
A sprinkling of Himalayan pink salt

Place everything in a bowl and use a hand mixer to blend to a smooth batter; alternatively, use a blender, for example a NutriBullet.

Using a ceramic pan you don't need any oil – just heat the pan to medium/warm heat.

Spoon ¼ cup of batter per pancake into the pan.

Turn the heat to medium low.

Cook for a couple of minutes until the pancake has firmed up, then carefully flip it over and cook for another few minutes until it has a beautiful, golden colour on the other side too.

Serve with fresh berries, maple syrup, coconut yoghurt, organic jam, fresh fruit – whatever you love.

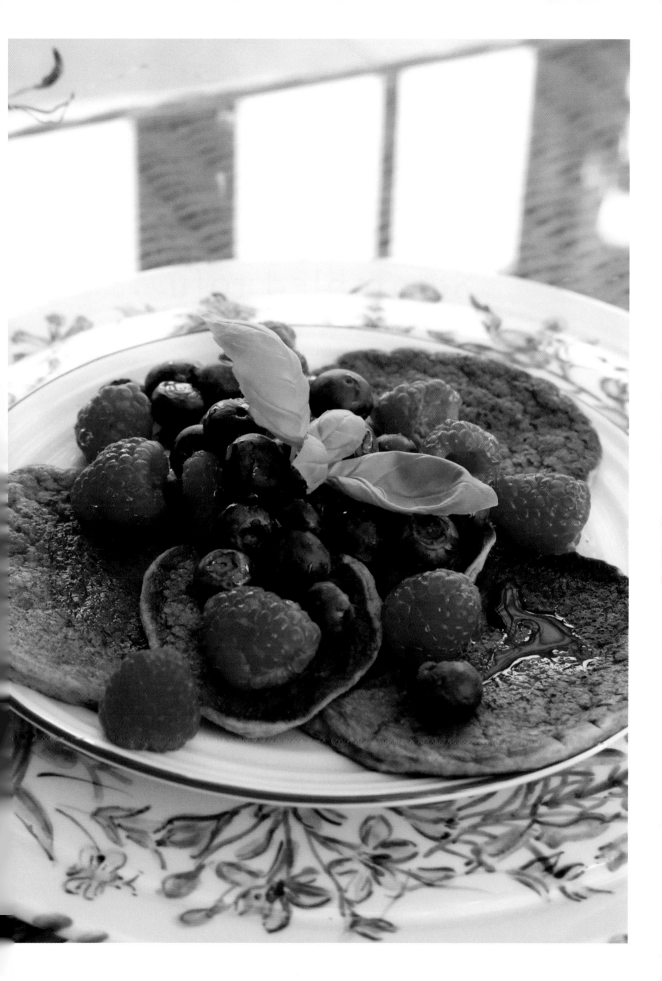

Tofu

Scrambled tofu

Silken tofu falls apart into a lovely scramble and the sauce gives
it all a gorgeous, bright yellow colour.

SERVES: 2-3

300 g silken tofu
1 shallot, chopped
1 clove of garlic, minced
Sauce
2 tbsp nutritional yeast
¼ tsp turmeric
¼ tsp organic herb salt
¼ tsp paprika
Black pepper
2 tbsp filtered water

Serve with:
Garlic-infused spinach
(page 152)
Cherry tomatoes
Oven-roasted potatoes
or sweet potatoes

The best way to cook silken tofu I find is to drain it
before cooking. Empty the contents of the tofu package
into a fine mesh sieve which is suspended above a small
bowl. Then use another bowl to press down on the tofu
so the water is squeezed out and collects in the bowl
underneath. Leave to drain for 15 minutes.

Mix all the sauce ingredients in a mug and keep
this to hand.

Heat a dash of water in a frying pan, turn the heat
down to medium and add the shallot and garlic. Cook
for a few minutes until translucent and keep adding
water so the mixture doesn't stick to the pan.

Add the tofu and break it up with a spatula, but do
leave a few chunks.

Allow the tofu mixture to warm up, and stir
occasionally for about a minute; then pour in the sauce
and mix well. Once warm, turn off the heat.

I usually serve the scrambled tofu with cherry tomatoes
warmed in a pan, garlic-infused spinach (page 152) and
oven-roasted potatoes or sweet potatoes.

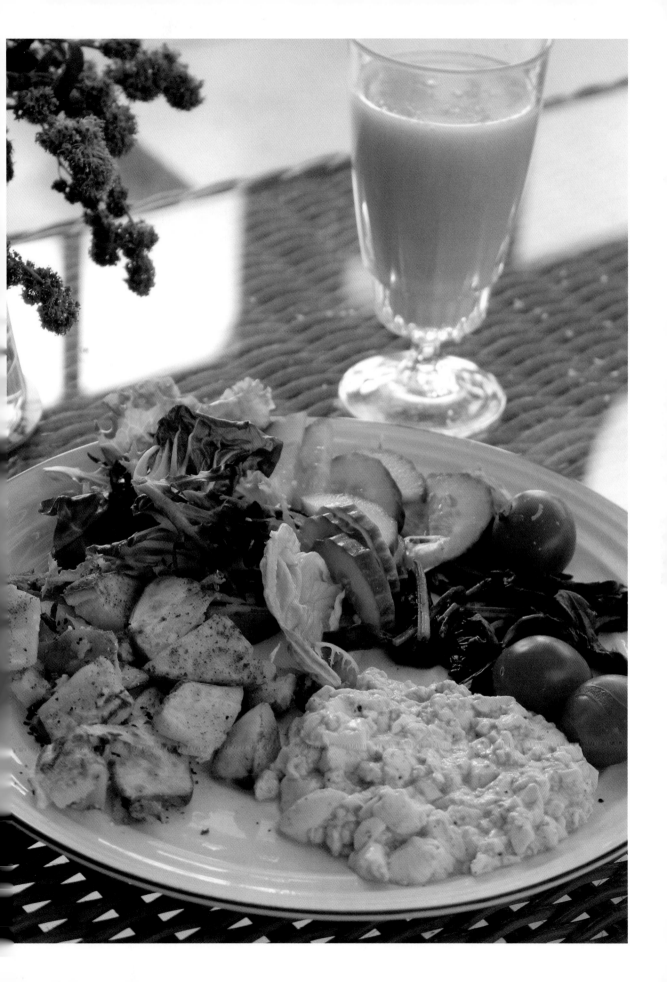

Early morning porridge toppings

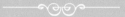

Blueberry compote

Raw blueberries are little powerhouses of nutrients but sometimes it is nice to have them warm, so here is a lovely blueberry compote to top off your winter porridge.

1 cup blueberries
2 tbsp water

Place your blueberries and the water in a pot on the stove and heat until the berries are close to boiling. At that point turn the heat off - do not bring to the boil in order to retain nutrients.

Serve over porridge.

Apple sauce

Choose organic apples, give them a good wash and leave the skin on as it contains excellent fibre, vitamins and other micro-nutrients, including the antioxidant quercetin.

3 apples, chopped
½ tsp lemon juice
1 cup water
½ tsp cinnamon
¼ tsp of maple syrup
- optional

Place the apples, lemon juice and water in a saucepan and bring to the boil.

Boil on a low heat for 20 minutes, until soft.

Mash it all up with a fork, hand-blender or potato masher and stir in the cinnamon. If you find that it is a bit sour, just stir in ¼ tsp of maple syrup.

Serve on top of your favourite porridge or use in desserts as an oil replacement.

Lasts up to a week in the fridge in an airtight container.

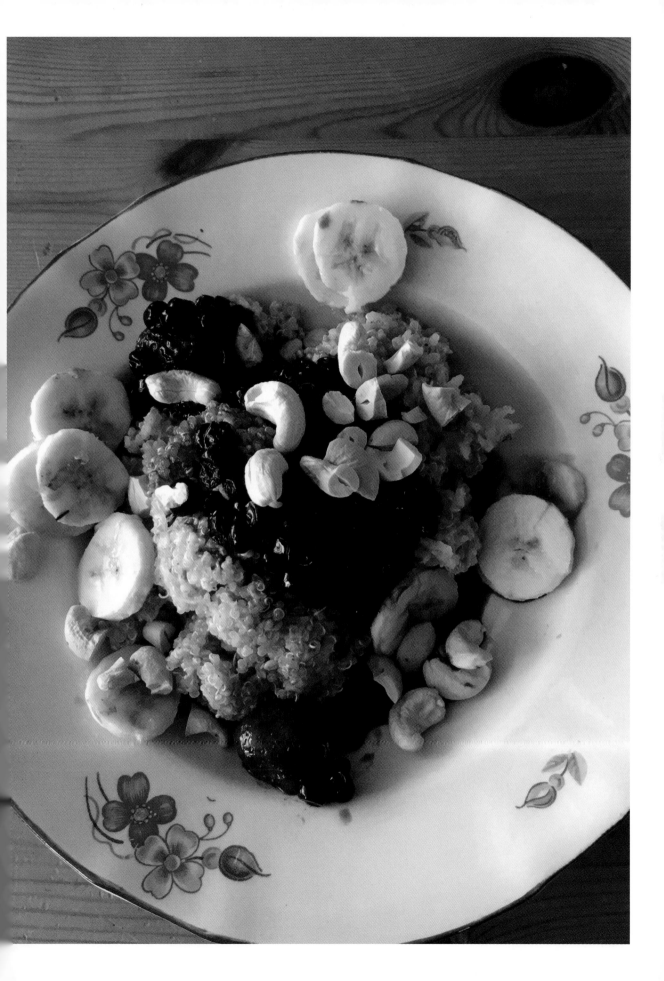

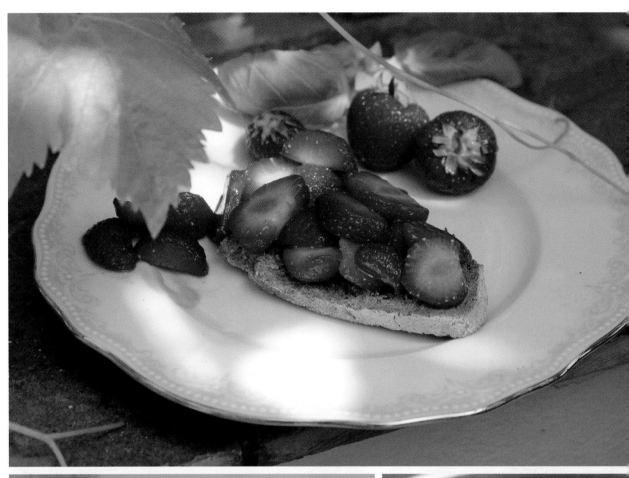

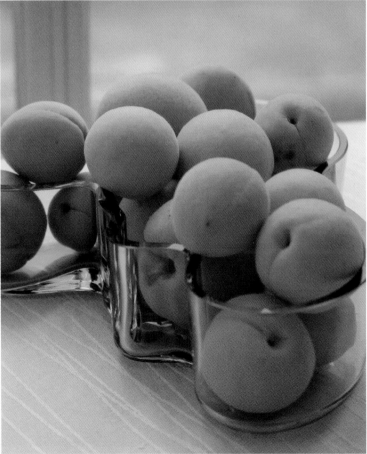

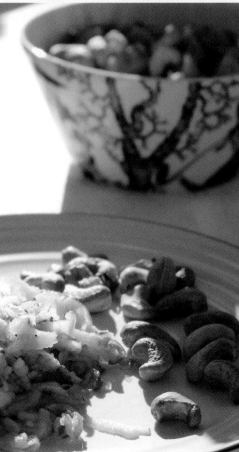

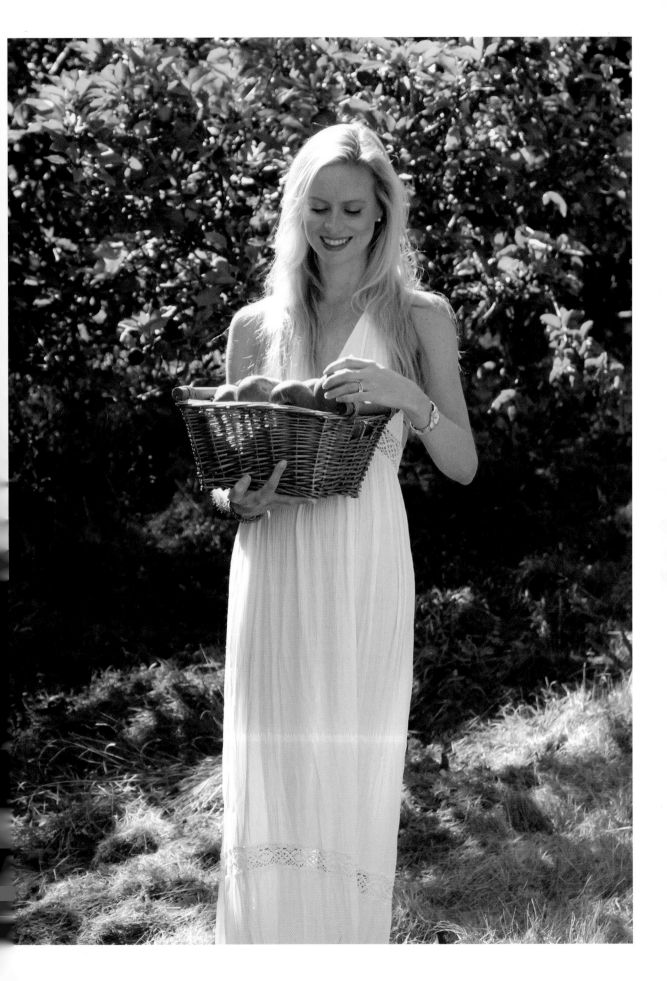

Raw strawberry compote

By keeping the strawberries raw you retain all their nutrients and goodness, so this is a lovely alternative to the cooked version. This compote is also delicious on toast.

1 cup strawberries
½ tsp maple syrup

Slice the strawberries and place in a bowl.

Drizzle the maple syrup over and stir for a minute.

Leave to rest for half an hour to get the consistency of a compote before serving on top of toasted spelt bread, or on a gluten-free bread of your choice.

Strawberry jam

3 cups of chopped strawberries
½ cup of water
1 tbsp blackstrap molasses

Combine all the ingredients in a saucepan, boil on a low heat for a maximum of 20 minutes, stirring occasionally.

When the consistency is to your liking, the jam is done. For thicker jam, just let it cook for longer.

This strawberry jam is lovely on top of porridge and it is also the best topping for the Christmassy rice porridge (page 40).

Apricot jam

2 cups of fresh apricots, chopped
1 cup of water
2 tbsp maple syrup
1 tbsp chia seeds

In a saucepan bring the apricots, water and maple syrup to the boil, then turn the heat to medium and boil for about 10 minutes until the apricots are soft.

The sweetness of the jam depends on how ripe the apricots are, so do feel free to add more maple syrup if it is not quite sweet enough for your liking, and less if the apricots are already very sweet

Turn the heat off and mash the apricots with a fork or a potato masher.

Stir in the chia seeds.

Pour the jam into a glass jar and allow to cool before serving.

Delicious when smeared on toast or served on top of porridge.

Store in the fridge, where it lasts about a week. However, it is so delicious that you might just end up eating it within a couple of days!

Dry-roasted cashews

Raw, organic cashew nuts

Soaking the cashews in filtered water overnight makes them easier to digest but leaving them unsoaked gives them more crunch in this specific recipe – test and see what works best for you.

Preheat the oven to 175°C or 350°F (Mark 4).

Spread the cashews on a baking tray lined with baking parchment.

Place in the oven for 12 minutes, then take them out and allow to cool for 10 minutes. They will keep sizzling away for a little while after they have come out of the oven.

Eat them sprinkled on top of your porridge, in a salad or scattered on top of your stir-fry or in the summer rolls (page 80). Eating leafy greens or a green smoothie at the same time will make them more digestible.

Toast toppings

So, without meat, cheese and butter, what goes on toast?

I have found local food markets to be great places to find freshly baked, oil-free bread. My favourite is a spelt sourdough loaf which is seriously delicious; spelt is not gluten free, but its gluten structure is slightly different to that of wheat and for me it has worked very well, so I always keep slices of it in the freezer, which are great when toasted. This is something to test for yourself to see how it makes you, personally, feel.

Finnish sourdough rye bread is another favourite and I bring loads back to the UK from Sweden and Finland every time I visit. Some Scandinavian cafes in London serve it too, so do try it if you get the chance.

Brown rice miso paste

A smearing of brown rice miso paste is delicious on toast and can be further topped with lettuce and other veggies for a super-nutritious snack.

Hummus

I love making my own hummus (see page 157) as it is so quick and can be varied endlessly. Often hummus recipes contain tahini, but as mentioned previously, the higher fat content then makes it quite an advanced food if you have rheumatoid arthritis. Luckily the tahini can be left out without compromising on flavour or texture.

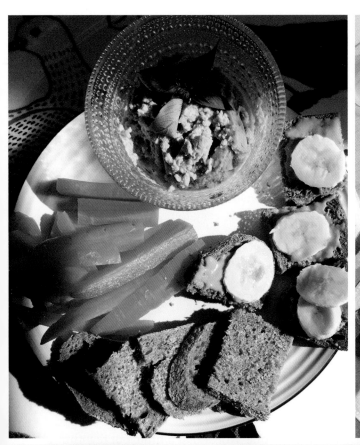
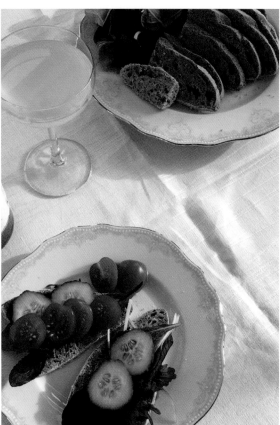
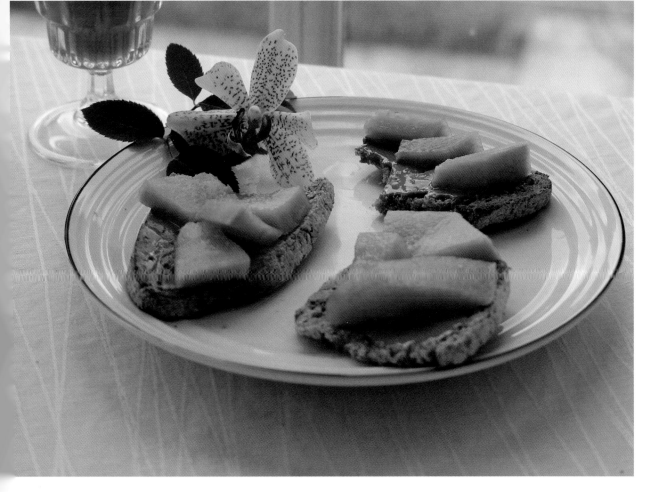

Tahini

Tahini (sesame seed butter) is delicious on toast but owing to the high fat content is quite an advanced food and it took me about a year and a half before I started having it. Initially, I would always have it with a side salad or some spinach leaves to help my gut break it down. Now that I can enjoy it, a sound favourite is tahini and sliced banana on toast, but it is also lovely with melon, avocado or raw veggies. Toast your bread, smear on some tahini, line up your toppings and enjoy. It is also the perfect take-away snack, easy to pack and filling while you are on the go.

Avocado

Due to my body's inability to break down fats with the inflammatory arthritis, it took me about nine months to be able to tolerate avocados again. Yes, that was sad, but with all the small improvements that I noticed every day I didn't mourn the loss too long - you get a very good perspective on life when you get hit by an illness like this.

These days I am still careful and only have about ¼ of one avocado at a time, but few things are better than smashed avocado on toast with black pepper, a sprinkling of Himalayan pink salt and a squeeze of lemon. I usually also have a big handful of fresh baby spinach on the side as this helps me digest the fat.

Nut butters

Nut butters are another more advanced topping, again due to the higher fat content, so just be patient if you are on the Paddison Program and you will eventually get to these beauties. They are perfect on toast: just smear some almond, cashew or peanut butter on toast and top it all off with some yummy veggies - for example, cucumber, cocktail tomatoes, gem lettuce and radishes or sliced banana.

Strawberry compote

In the Early morning porridge toppings on page 54, you will find the delicious Raw strawberry compote that is yummy on toast, especially with a cup of fresh mint tea on the side.

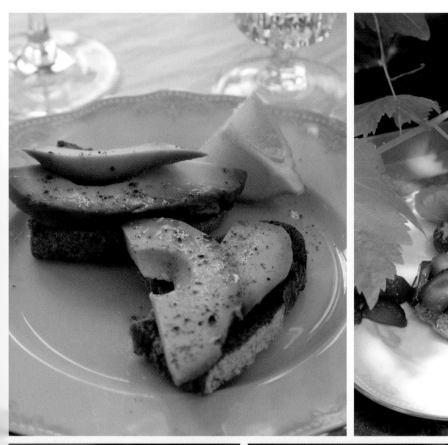
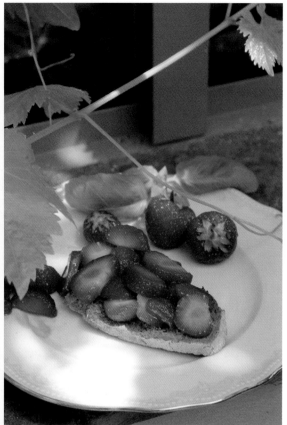
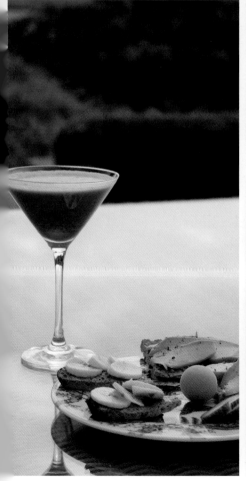
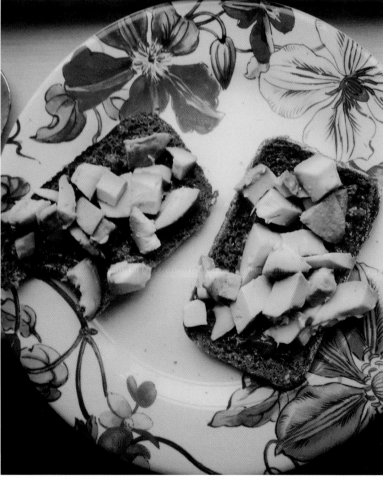

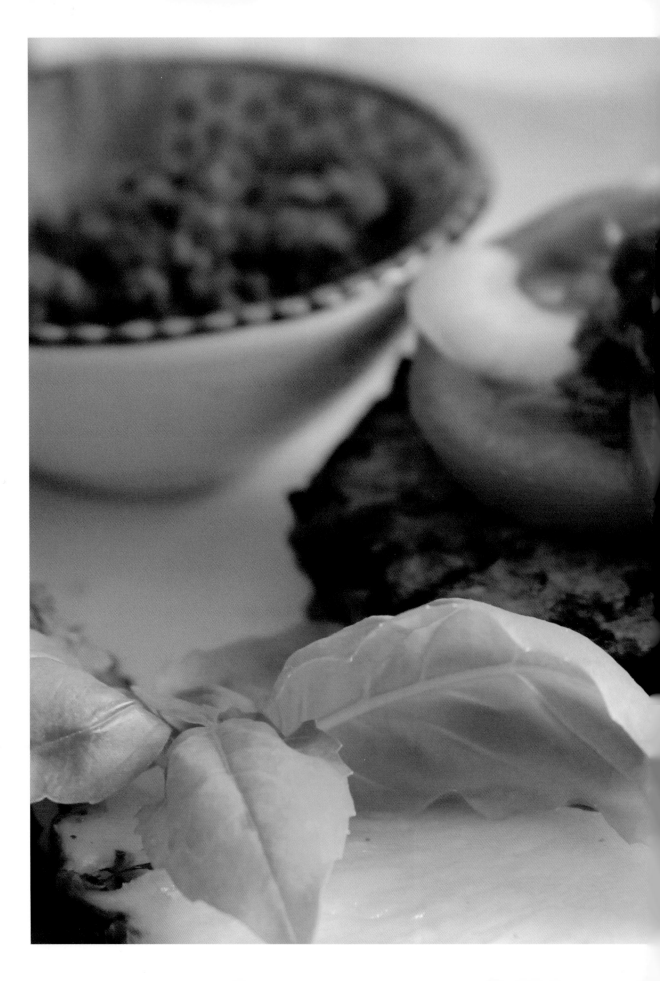

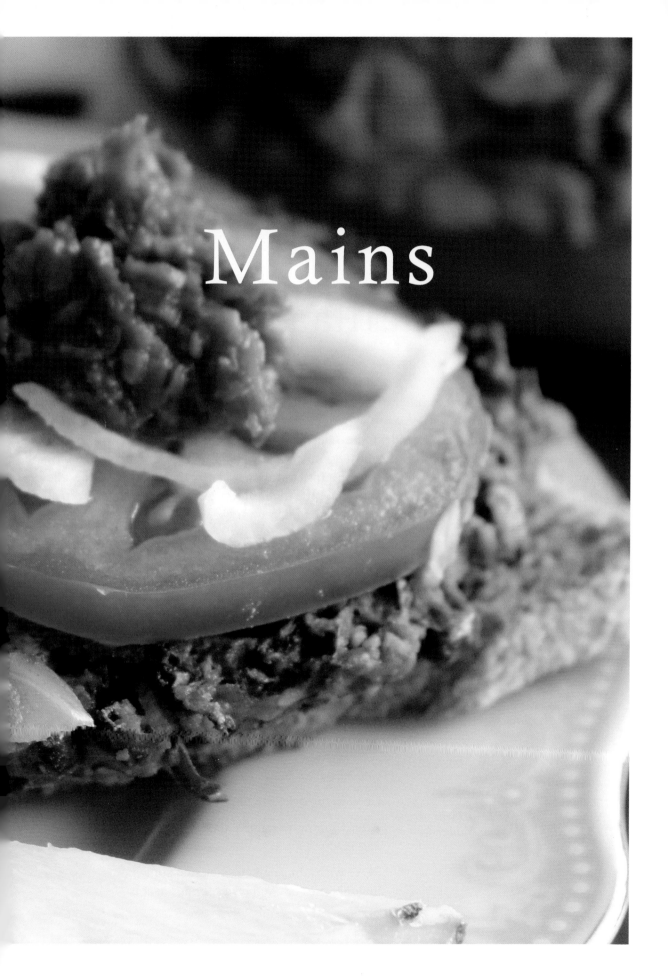

Mains

Rice dishes

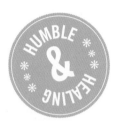

Kaalilaatikko
Finnish cabbage delight

This was one of the first familiar dishes that I was able to have after starting the Paddison Program. It is delicious yet kind to the system and you can increase the calorie intake by having boiled potatoes on the side. Once you can tolerate more foods, do feel free to add other spices and veggies – this is the most humble version. I know it may sound odd to have both potatoes and rice in a dish but some Finnish families swear by the potatoes on the side, and some would never have it that way. I suppose the need for extra starches stems from all those freezing mid-winter evenings!

SERVES: 4

1 onion, diced
1 clove of garlic, minced
½ cabbage, shredded
2 carrots, cubed
2 tsp Tamari sauce
1 cup Basmati rice
1 tsp Himalayan pink salt
2½ cups of water
2 tsp maple syrup – optional

Optional to serve with:
Boiled potatoes
Lingonberries or cranberries

Preheat the oven to 220°C or 425°F (Mark 7).

In a ceramic saucepan, steam-fry the onion and garlic in a dash of water until soft.

Add the cabbage and carrots and let it all fuse together for another few minutes.

Pour in the Tamari sauce and rice, cover with boiling hot water and mix well; turn off the heat.

Transfer the mixture into a non-stick, oven-proof dish, ideally one with a lid.

Optional: drizzle the maple syrup over the top.

Cook in the oven for 10 minutes.

After 10 minutes remove the lid, or until the rice is soft and ready.

Serve with a huge green salad and some raw lingonberries or cranberries, or just as it is.

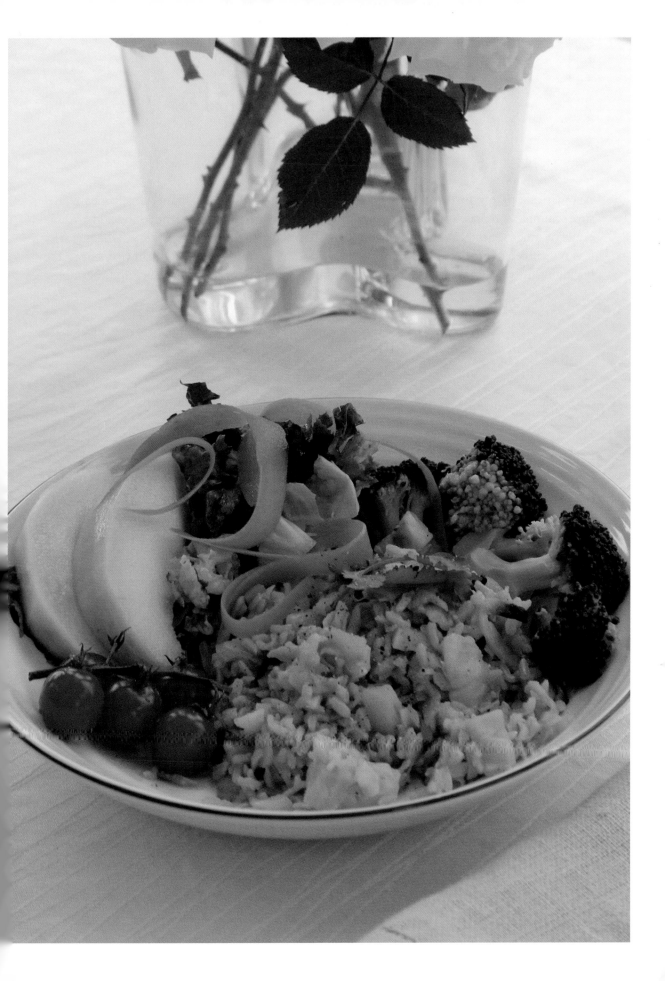

Super-humble sushi rolls

Another one of my first 'real' dishes after joining the Paddison Program, which means it is super-humble and once your system gets more robust you can get more creative and add a whole range of other vegetables. I could only tolerate Basmati rice for the longest time, which is why it is my choice of rice in this recipe. I know it doesn't stick together like sushi rice, but in the beginning my priority was to get the sushi flavours of the nori, rice, Tamari sauce and vegetables.

2-3 nori sheets
1 cup Basmati rice, cooked and cooled down
½ cucumber, cut into thin strips
1 carrot, cut into thin strips or grated

Any other favourite vegetables:
Alfalfa sprouts
Mung bean sprouts
Avocado, cut into thin strips
Cabbage, cut into thin strips

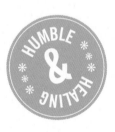

Place the nori sheet on a dry cutting board or a sushi mat.

Spread the rice on top of the sheet, leaving approximately 1 cm at the end.

Line up your vegetables in single rows on top of the rice.

Roll the nori sheet away from you so the vegetables are folded into the centre.

Slice the roll into six pieces with a wet knife.

Dip into Tamari sauce with a side of brown rice miso soup (page 137) with torn seaweed and sliced spring onion.

You can also make your own wasabi paste using wasabi powder and warm water if you wish to avoid the additives that are often found in the ready-made wasabi.

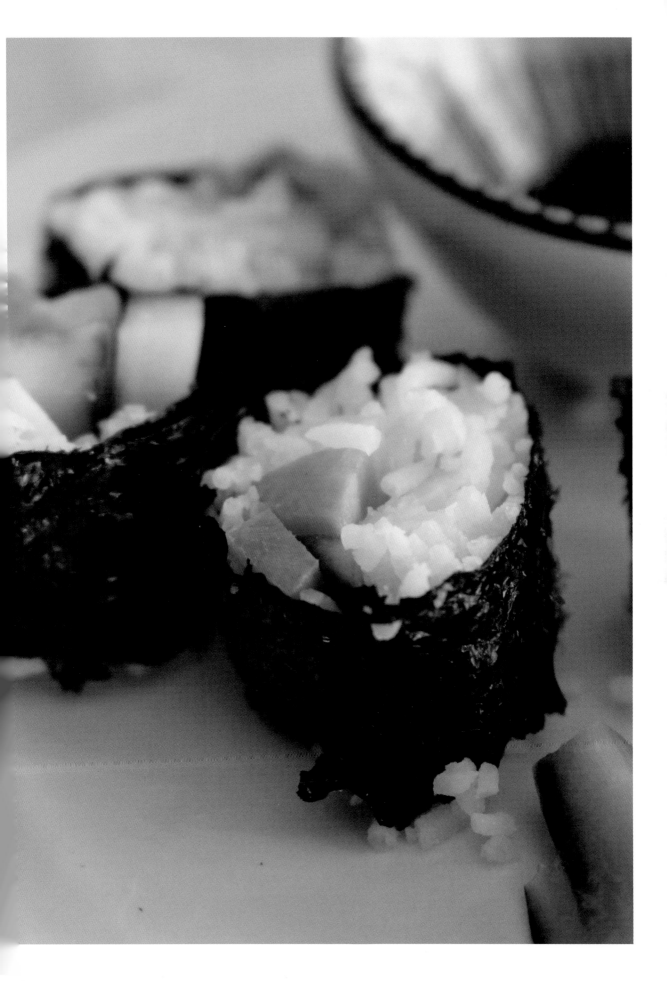

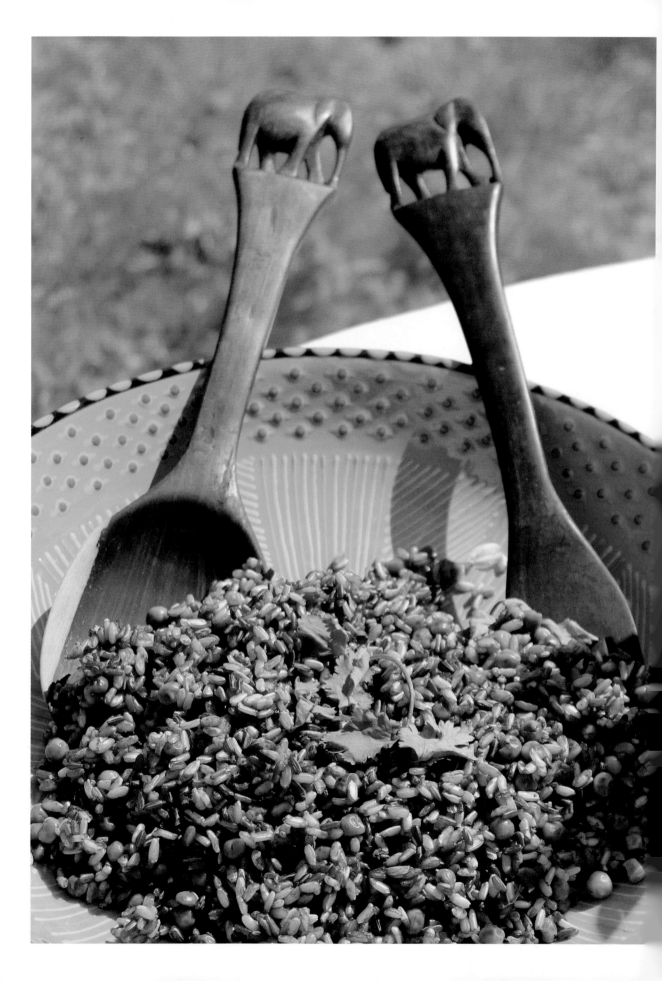

Wild rice risotto

This is a wonderful recipe that can be made with any veggies that you can tolerate: courgette, butternut squash, broccoli etc. I love the excuse to get more veggies into the dish and just steam them before adding to the rice. As always on a plant-based diet, it is hard to say how many portions this results in, as you will just eat until you are satisfied, but 2-3 is a good guide.

SERVES: 2-3

1 cup wild rice
1 cup frozen peas
½ cup filtered water
2 cups sliced mushrooms
2 tsp Tamari sauce
Black pepper
Himalayan pink salt or
Organic herb salt

Cook the rice as per the instructions on the packet.

With five minutes left of the cooking time, stir in the peas and allow to finish cooking together.

Heat a sprinkling of the water in a ceramic pan and scatter in the mushrooms. Let them cook away on medium heat until they have wilted. Season the mushrooms with the Tamari sauce, black pepper and salt or Herbamare.

Slowly add the rest of the water and let it infuse with the mixture, so that you get a stock.

Mix the mushrooms and stock with the rice, peas and serve.

Apple and beetroot risotto

This risotto can be made in two ways – with or without the beetroot – so you get either a delicious apple and beetroot risotto or an amazing apple risotto.

SERVES: 4

1 large beetroot, peeled and cut into small chunks
2 cloves garlic
1 yellow onion, chopped
400 grams Arborio rice
1 litre of vegetable broth (see page 136)
(You can use shop-bought stock but it usually contains oils so I would warmly recommend spending an hour making your own big batch, as you can freeze the leftover broth and use it in other dishes.)
1 apple, diced
Juice from ½ lemon

Preheat the oven to 200°C or 400°F (Mark 6).

Put the beetroot and the garlic clove on parchment paper in the middle of the oven and roast for 30 minutes, until soft.

In a large ceramic pan, steam-fry the onion and one clove of minced garlic in a dash of water until soft.

Stir in the rice, then add ½ cup of the veggie broth. Stir well and cook until the rice has soaked up the broth.

Add the diced apple and lemon juice, mix and pour in 1 cup of broth. Turn to a low heat.

Keep stirring until the rice has absorbed the broth, then add another cup of broth.

Keep adding the broth, one cup at the time, until all has been absorbed. Make sure to stir often so that the rice does not stick to the bottom of the pan.

Once the beetroot is cooked, place it in a blender with a dash of water and blend until you have a paste – it doesn't need to be completely smooth.

Mix the beetroot into the risotto.

Check seasoning and add some Himalayan pink salt to taste, or Herbamare spice.

Serve and enjoy.

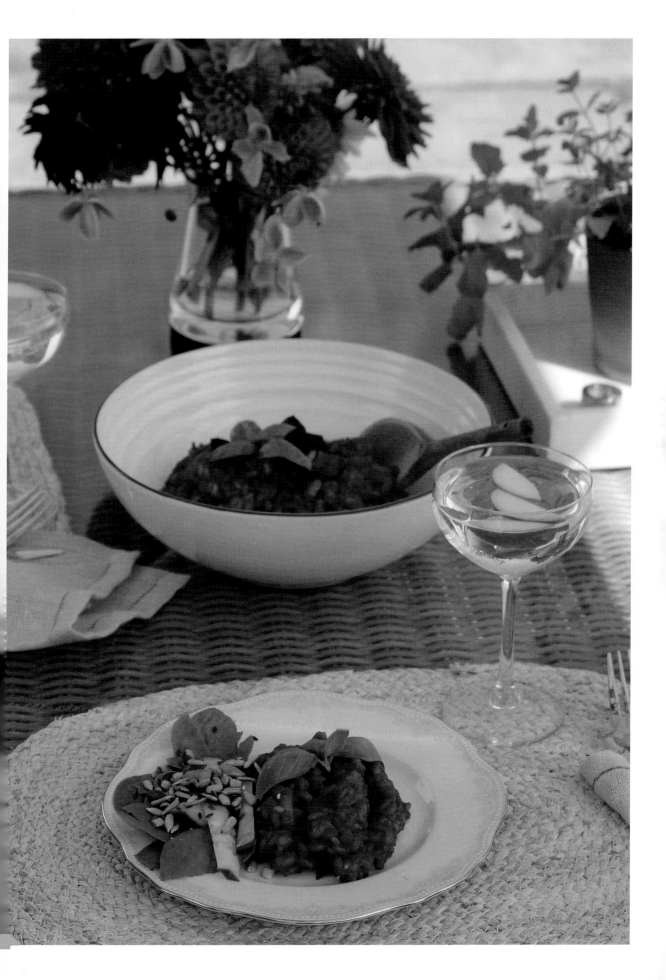

Stuffed tomatoes

SERVES: 2

Two large beef tomatoes
1 onion, chopped
1 clove garlic, minced
Himalayan pink salt
Black pepper
A dash of cayenne
pepper – optional
1 can organic black beans,
rinsed, or ½ cup black beans,
soaked overnight and cooked
as per the instructions on the
package
1 handful fresh spinach
1 tsp Tamari sauce
1 cup white or brown
Basmati rice
Fresh coriander
Water, filtered

Preheat the oven to 200°C or 400°F (Mark 6).

Carefully cut out the top of the tomato, like a lid, and set aside.

Spoon out the insides of the tomato and place in a bowl.

In a ceramic saucepan, steam-fry the onions and garlic in a little water until soft, then add the tomato, salt, pepper and spices.

Add the black beans, spinach leaves and Tamari sauce to the onions – warm but do not bring to the boil.

Stuff the tomatoes with the bean stew and place the tomato lids on top of each tomato.

Cook in the oven for 20 minutes.

Meanwhile, cook the Basmati rice.

Serve the tomatoes with the rice and a large green salad on the side.

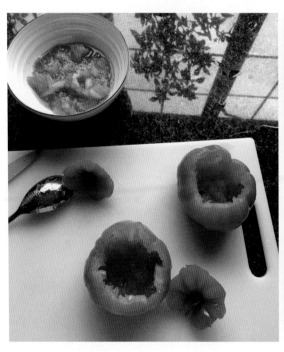
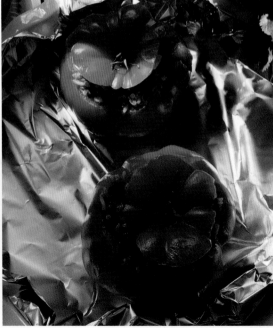

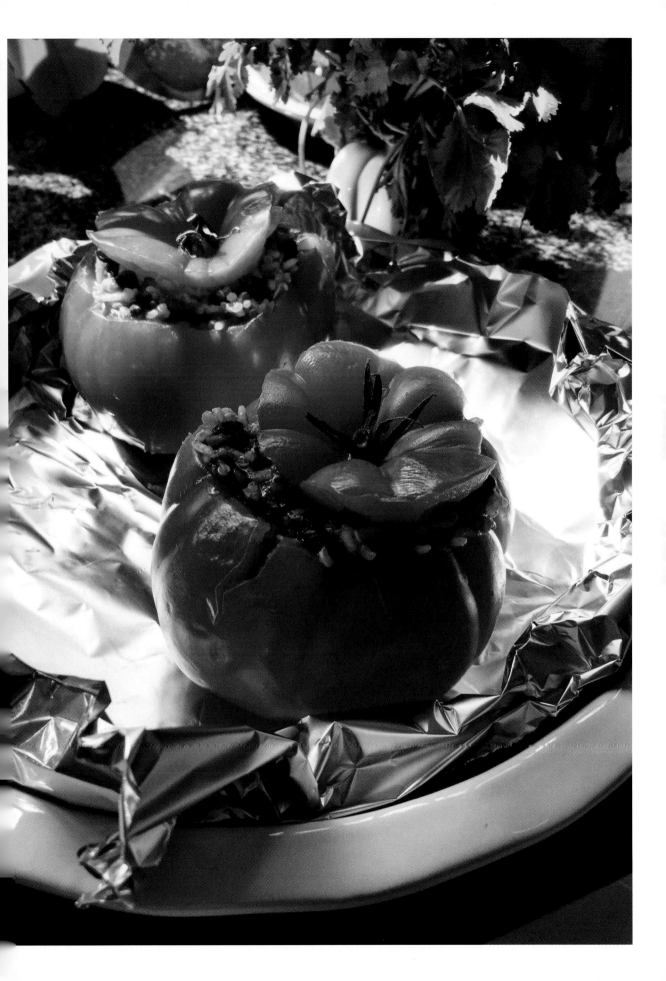

Mushroom and aubergine stroganoff

SERVES: 4

1 onion, chopped
2 cups of aubergine, chopped
2 cups of mushrooms, chopped
2 tsp Tamari sauce
Himalayan pink salt, to taste
Black pepper
½ tsp paprika
½ tsp white pepper
3 tomatoes, blended in a blender
½ cup oat milk or nut milk
2 tsp gluten-free flour
⅙ cup cold filtered water

Serve with:
1½ cup brown Basmati rice

In a ceramic saucepan, steam-fry the onion in a dash of water until translucent.

Add another sprinkling of water, the aubergine and mushrooms and cook until soft.

Add the seasoning, the tomatoes and the nut milk and stir well.

In a mug, stir the gluten-free flour into the cold water until you have a smooth paste.

Stir the flour mix into the sauce to thicken it, and keep stirring until you are happy with the consistency.

Serve with brown Basmati rice and, of course a lovely big green salad on the side.

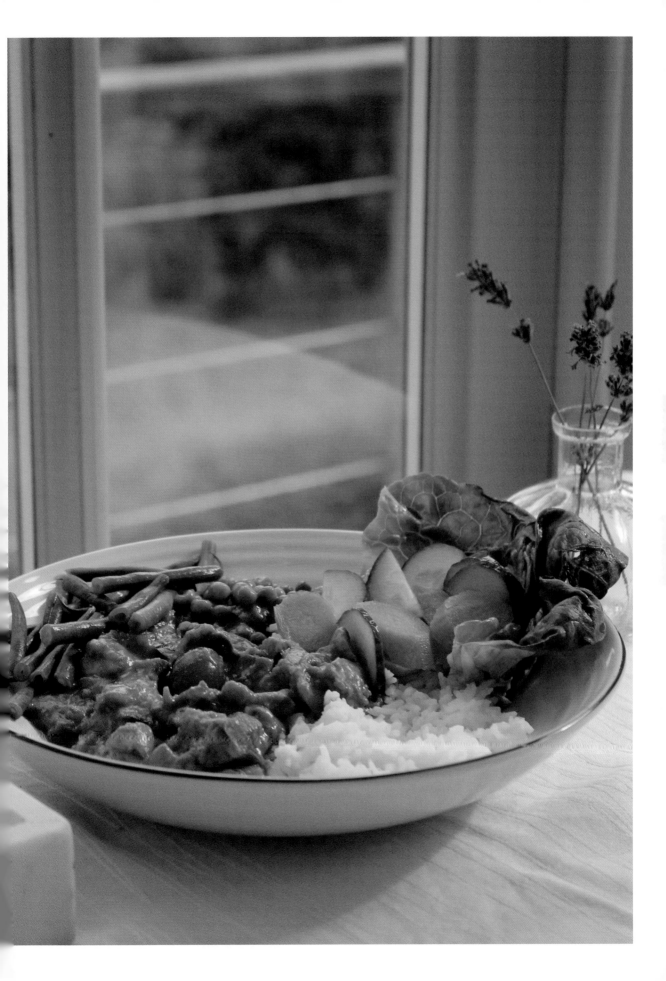

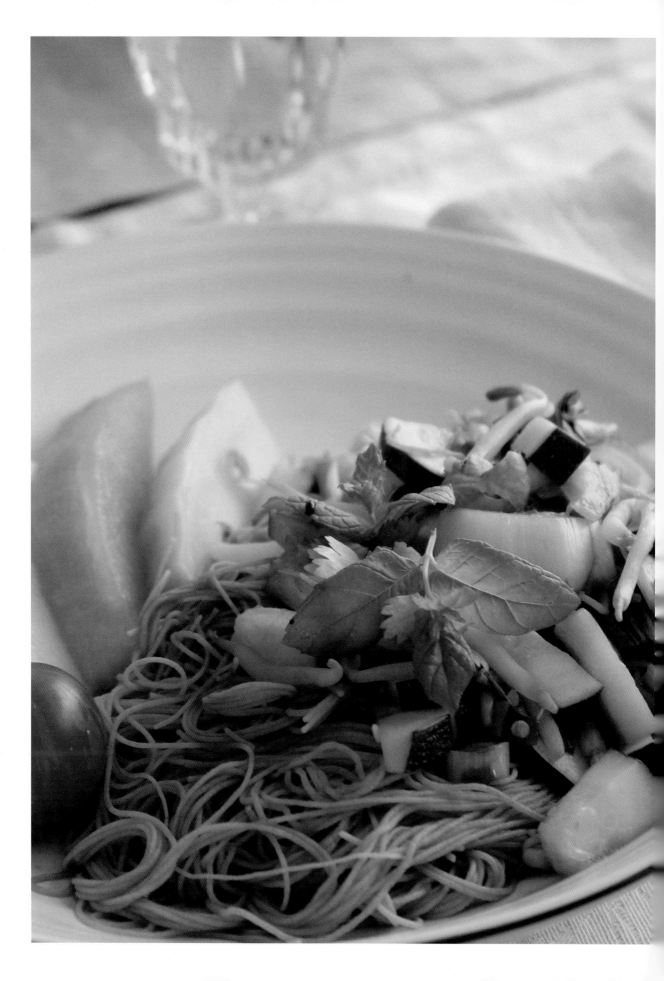

Noodles and summer rolls

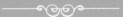

Stir-fries and summer rolls are just the best, as you can vary the vegetables endlessly and create the most mouth-watering combinations.

With stir-fries the key is cooking the vegetables so that they retain their crunch, as this will help preserve their nutrients.

These ingredients make up a great flavour-base for stir-fries: garlic, fresh ginger, fresh chillies, Tamari sauce, lime or lemon.

Courgette stir-fry

SERVES: 2

Serve with:
2 nests of rice noodles

Stir-fry:
*1 clove garlic, minced
1 small fresh red chilli pepper,
chopped
3 cm fresh ginger, chopped finely
2 cups mushrooms, sliced
1 courgette, halved then cut into
half moons
1 bok choy, sliced
Tamari sauce
½ lime*

Cook the rice noodles according to the instructions on the packet.

In a ceramic wok (or large saucepan) steam-fry the garlic, chilli and ginger in a dash of water for 30 seconds.

Add the mushrooms and cook for a couple of minutes until they start getting a bit of colour. Add more water if needed.

Add the courgette and bok choy and cook for a minute, until all the vegetables are heated through but not too soft.

Add a splash of Tamari sauce, stir well.

Turn off the heat and pour in the noodles.

Squeeze the lime on top and mix well.

Enjoy!

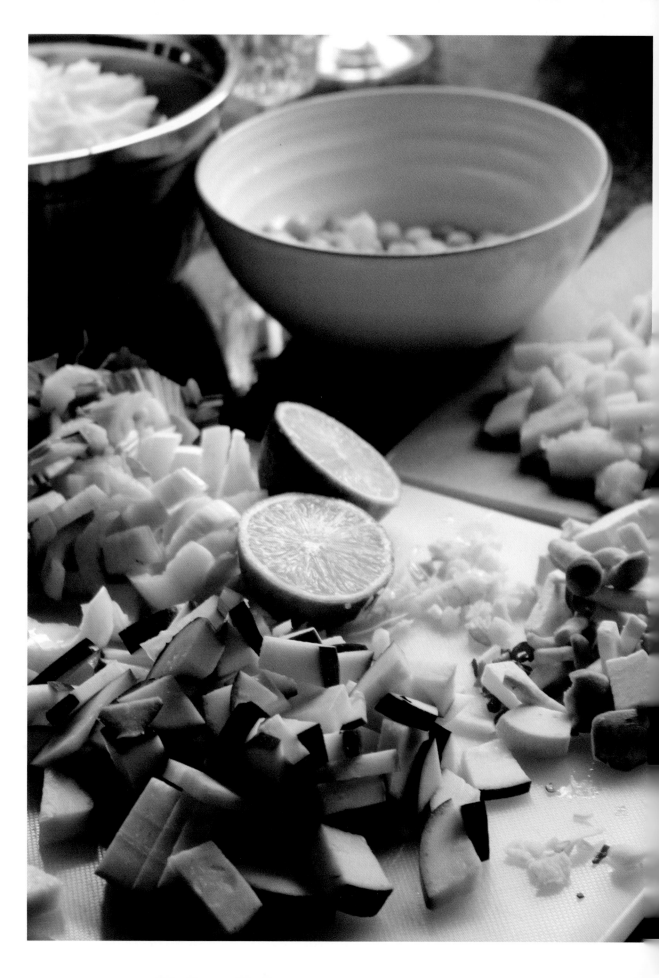

The fridge-emptying stir-fry

This is the perfect recipe for using up whatever bits and bobs you have lying around in the fridge. Half an aubergine and three carrots? Some partly dried mint and coriander? Chop it up and chuck it all in – and herbs are absolutely fine to use even if they look dry and sad as they still taste delicious.

SERVES: 2

Serve with:
*2 nests of rice noodles
or 1 cup Basmati rice*

Stir-fry:
*½ cauliflower,
cut into very small florets
1 clove garlic, minced
1 small fresh red chilli
pepper, chopped
3 cm fresh ginger, chopped finely
½ cabbage, sliced finely
1 courgette, halved then
sliced into half-moons
A large handful of
spinach, rinsed
Pomegranate seeds
Dry-roasted cashew nuts
(page 55)*

Cook the noodles or rice according to the instructions on the packet.

Heat a ceramic wok or large pan and add a splash of water.

Add the cauliflower and cook until it starts to soften; keep adding water as needed.

Add the garlic, chilli and ginger, stir well and cook for one minute.

Add the cabbage and courgette and cook for another minute.

Finally, stir in the spinach and allow to wilt for a few seconds, then turn off the heat.

Serve with the noodles or rice, with the pomegranate seeds and cashews scattered on top.

Chickpea stir-fry

SERVES: 2

Serve with:
*2 nests of rice noodles
or 1 cup Basmati rice*

Stir-fry:
*1 clove garlic, minced
1 small fresh red chilli
pepper, chopped
3 cm fresh ginger, chopped
½ cabbage, shredded
1 large carrot, sliced thinly
2 large handfuls of
mushrooms, chopped or sliced
2 tsp Tamari sauce*

Chickpeas:
*½ can chickpeas, drained
or 1 cup chickpeas soaked
overnight and cooked as per the
instructions on the package
½ tsp cayenne pepper
Juice from ½ lemon
1 clove garlic, minced*

*Fresh coriander
Fresh mint leaves*

Cook the rice noodles or Basmati rice and divide between two bowls.

Heat a dash of water in a ceramic saucepan and add the garlic, chilli and ginger.

Steam-fry for two minutes, before adding the cabbage, carrots, mushrooms and Tamari sauce.

Stir well and cook until the mushrooms have wilted.

Place on top of the noodles in each bowl.

To cook the chickpeas, heat a pan containing a small sprinkling of filtered water and add the chickpeas, garlic and lemon; sprinkle the cayenne pepper over the top.

Cook for two minutes, then sprinkle the chickpeas on top of the stir-fry.

Add the fresh herbs over the top and enjoy.

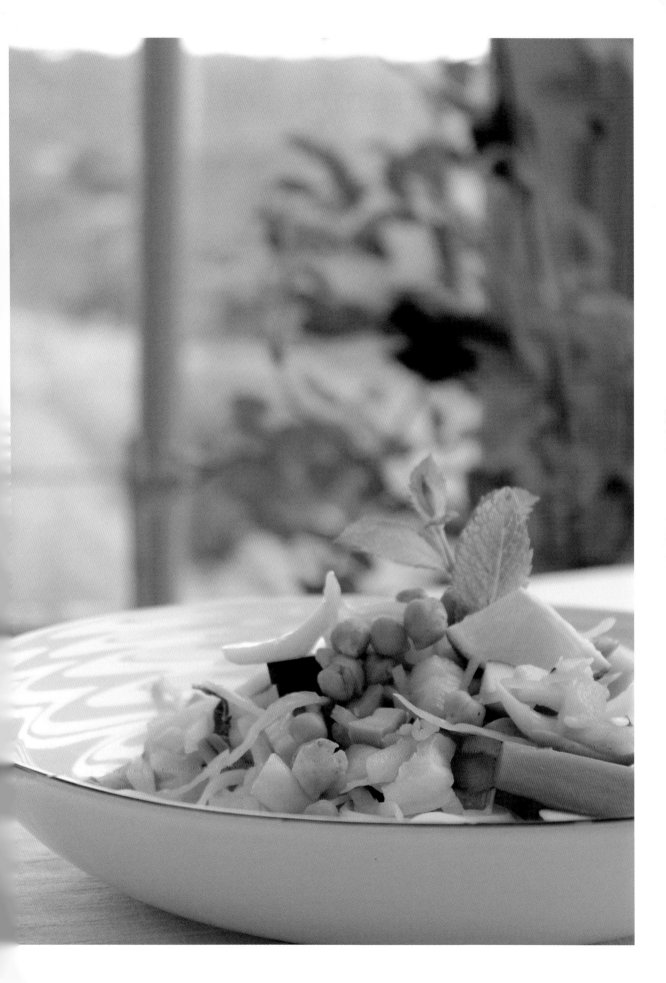

Summer rolls

Summer rolls are such crowd pleasers because everyone can stuff them with their favourite fresh veggies, fruits and nuts. The Spicy lime sauce and the Peanut sauce on the next page are perfect dips for these rolls.

Rice vermicelli noodles, cooked and cooled
Carrot, grated
Cucumber, cut into thin strips
Spring onion, cut into thin slices
Mango, cut into thin strips
Bean sprouts, rinsed
Tamari sauce
Fresh mint leaves
Rice paper
Dry-roasted cashew nuts, roughly chopped
Fresh, red chilli pepper, chopped finely
Fresh coriander leaves

Chop, cut and slice the carrot, cucumber, spring onion and mango – and other veggies of your choice – place them in separate bowls and make sure that you have approximately the same quantity of each.

Heat a saucepan containing a dash of water, add the rinsed bean sprouts and a quick shake of Tamari sauce, cook for about one minute. Set aside to cool.

Pick the leaves off the mint and place them in a bowl of cold water.

Boil a kettle of filtered water.

Have a large plate ready for your finished summer rolls and another, or a cutting board, for making them on.

Pour the boiled water onto a further large plate, for example a large pasta plate. Add a dash of cold water so you don't burn your fingers.

Dip the hard rice paper in the water on the plate, making sure that it gets fully submerged, and then place it flat on the clean plate, or cutting board. Once it has been soaked through it will keep getting softer so there is no need to soak for a long time.

Place some of your veggies and noodles in the middle of the paper, sprinkle over the chilli pepper, cashew nuts, the coriander and mint leaves.

Fold in the bottom, then the two sides on the right and the left so that they overlap, and finally the top, overlapping the rest.

Place the finished summer roll on the clean plate you have ready and move on to the next roll.

You can cut through them diagonally for a beautiful presentation but I usually just serve them whole.

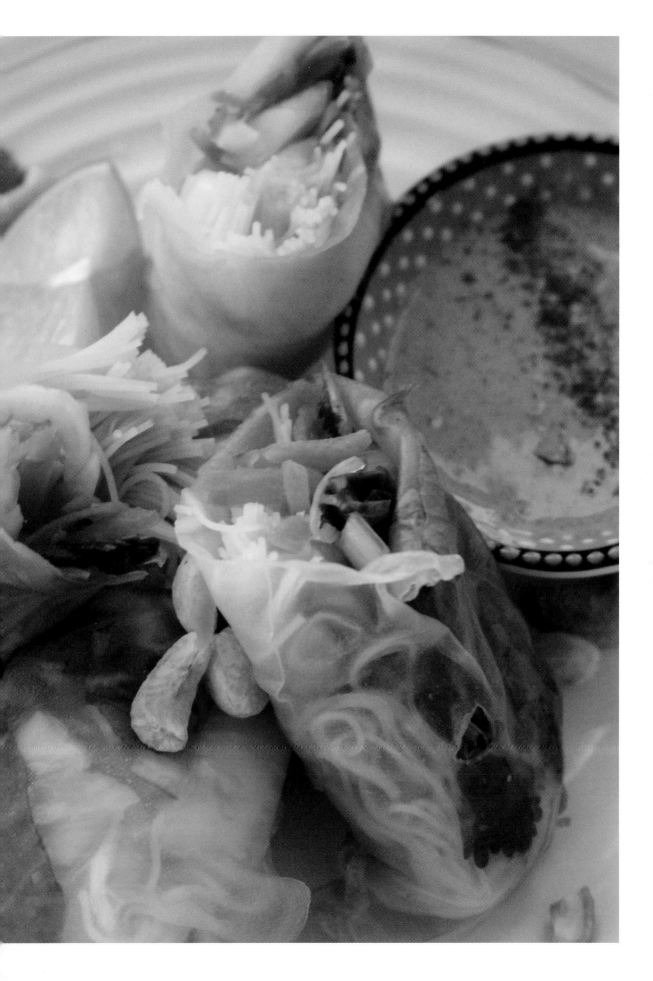

Spicy lime sauce

SERVES: 2

1 lime
*1 small fresh red chilli, deseeded
and finely chopped*
2 tsp Tamari sauce
1 tsp boiled water
1 tsp maple syrup
1 garlic clove, minced

Squeeze the lime juice
into a bowl.

Depending on how spicy
you like it, add half
or the whole deseeded chilli.

Stir in the rest of the ingredients.

The flavours infuse beautifully when the sauce is left
to sit at room temperature for an hour or more before
serving. It also keeps well in the fridge for about a
week.

Serve with the Summer rolls on page 80.

Peanut sauce

This sauce is just perfect with anything Thai-inspired, but it goes with so many other dishes
too. Choose a peanut butter made with only peanuts and nothing else. (Do remember to
check if any guests have allergies to peanuts, and this goes for other dishes with nuts, sesame
and celery too.)

4 tbsp peanut butter
*4 or 5 tbsp filtered water,
depending on how you thick you
want the sauce.*
*2 tbsp lemon juice
(approximately 1 lemon)*
3 tsp Tamari sauce
2 tsp maple syrup
*½ fresh bird's eye chilli; remove
the seeds for a less spicy version*
*A small handful of fresh
coriander leaves*

Add all the ingredients to a blender and blend until you
have a smooth sauce.

For a thicker sauce go for four tablespoons of water and
for a runnier sauce add five tablespoons.

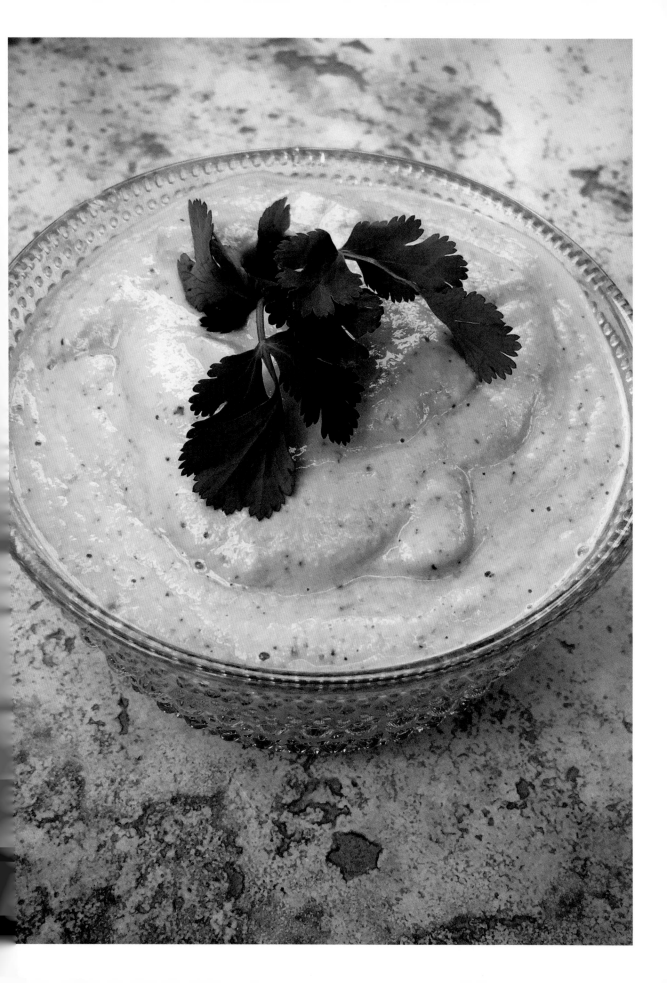

Pasta

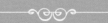

I cook mostly with gluten-free pasta; brown-rice, and corn-and-rice pasta have lovely flavour and consistency. Make sure the pasta isn't overcooked; it's better to have it a little bit *al dente*. To prevent the pasta from sticking after draining the cooking water, just rinse it a couple of times in cold water, tossing it between the sieve and the pot to cool it slightly. A sprinkling of boiled water just before serving will also help to unstick it.

Pasta and veggie delight

SERVES: 3-4

3 cups brown rice pasta
1 clove garlic, minced
2 cups butternut squash, cut into thin strips
½ cauliflower, cut into florets – optional
1 courgette, cut into thin strips
1 red onion, cut into chunks
1 can butter beans or ¼ cup soaked butter beans that you have cooked as per the instructions on the package – optional
Juice from ½ lemon
1 tsp Tamari sauce
Black pepper

Cook the pasta as per the instructions on the packet.

Heat a dash of water in a pan and add the garlic and butternut squash.

If you wish to include the cauliflower or any other of your favourite veggies, you can add them now.

Cook on medium heat until the butternut squash starts getting slightly soft; this can be anything from 5-15 minutes depending on the size of the strips. Keep adding water as needed to prevent the veggies from sticking to the pan.

Stir in the courgette and red onions and cook for another few minutes – the courgette should retain its crunch.

Stir in the butter beans here if you would like to include those.

Sprinkle with Tamari sauce and black pepper until you are happy with the seasoning.

Mix the veggies with the pasta and squeeze the lemon juice on top.

Serve and enjoy.

Some hummus (page 157) is also delicious with this.

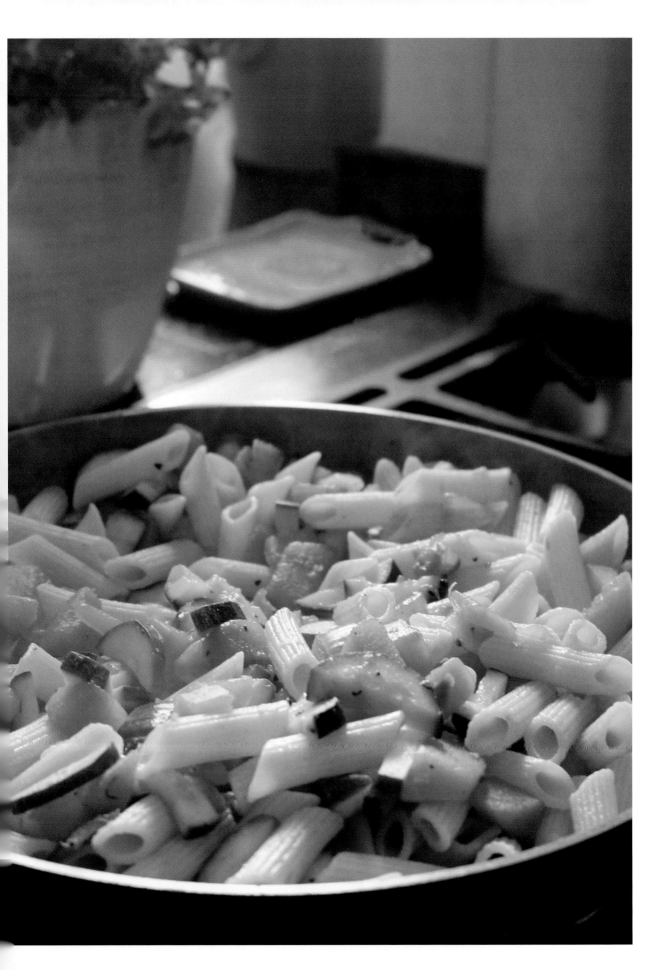

Spaghetti with a tomato and lentil ragu

This is such great comfort food – which in my world means food that is warm, nourishing, satisfying and leaves you feeling energised and awesome! Spaghetti and tomatoes are obviously always going to be a winning concept and it is so easy to alter old favourites into plant-based versions that taste just as wonderful.

SERVES: 4

1 onion, chopped
1 clove garlic, minced
1 can chopped tomatoes
200 grams red lentils
(approximately 1 cup), rinsed
1 cup carrots, grated
3 cups water
1 tsp dried mixed herbs
1 tsp dried oregano
2 bay leaves
Himalayan pink salt, to taste
1 tsp Tamari sauce
3 tsp balsamic vinegar
Black pepper
Gluten-free spaghetti
Fresh basil, leaves and stalks
separated, stalks chopped

In a ceramic saucepan steam-fry the onion and garlic in a dash of water until soft.

Add the rest of the ingredients, except for the basil leaves and spaghetti, bring to a boil, then turn the heat down and simmer for 45 minutes, or until the lentils are done.

If at this stage the sauce is too liquid, just turn up the heat to reduce it to your liking.

Cook the pasta and serve everything with fresh basil leaves scattered on top.

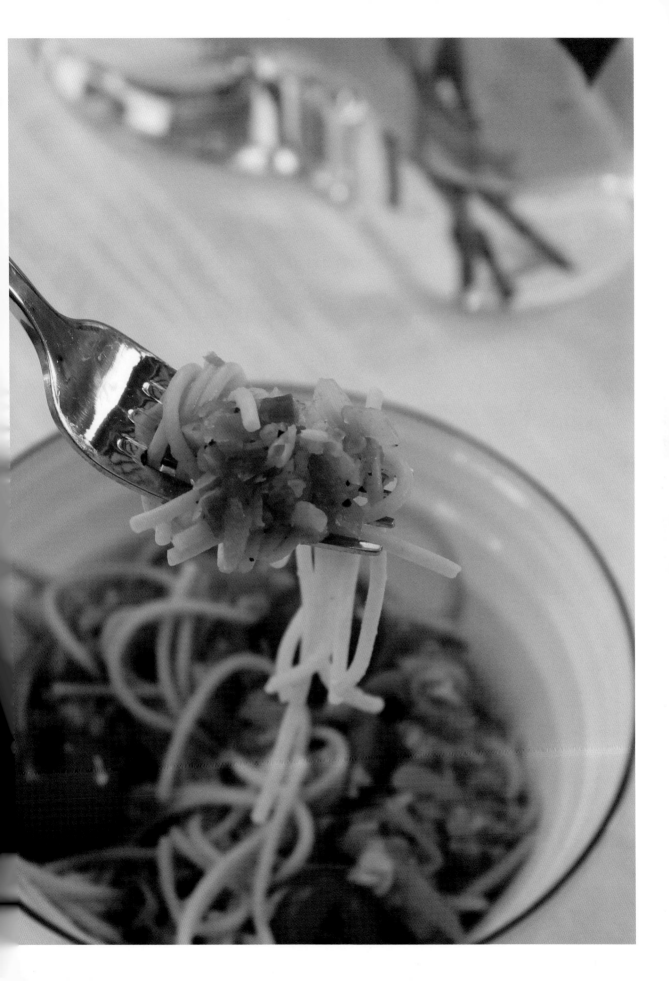

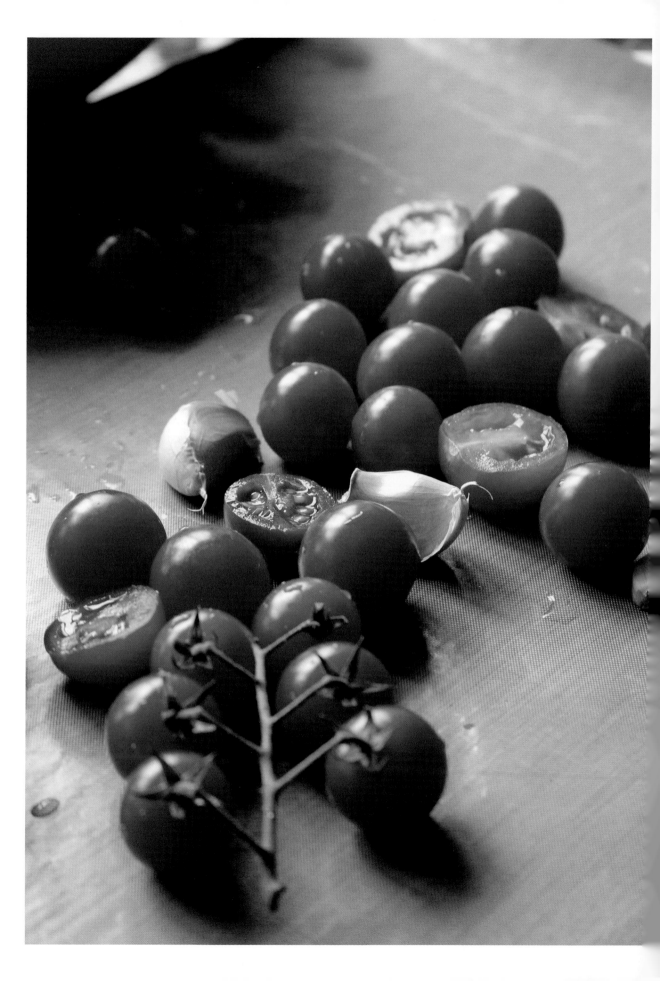

Pasta with a quick raw tomato sauce

Shop-bought ready-chopped tomatoes often contain additional ingredients, such as preservatives, not just tomatoes. When I initially started incorporating foods in my diet after the elimination part of the Paddison Program, I wanted to have foods that were as clean and whole as possible, which is why I used cocktail tomatoes instead of ready-chopped tomatoes. The result is a fresh and flavoursome tomato sauce.

SERVES: 2

20 cocktail tomatoes
A handful of basil leaves
Juice from ½ lemon
Black pepper, a few twists
Himalayan pink salt or organic herb salt, to taste
Brown rice pasta
2 tbsp nutritional yeast (optional, to give added nutritional value)

Cook the pasta as per the instructions on the packet.

Place the tomatoes in a blender whole together with the rest of the ingredients apart from the nutritional yeast if you choose to include that.

Blend until you have a smooth consistency – it is fine to have a few chunky bits of tomato left.

Stir in the nutritional yeast at this stage. Check seasoning

Stir the sauce into your pasta and enjoy!

This sauce can also be warmed in a saucepan before adding to the pasta – just make sure to turn off the heat before it starts boiling to retain as many of the nutrients as possible.

The sauce can be served with:

Oven-roasted vegetables (see recipe below)

6 artichoke hearts and 3 tbsp of capers, stirred in

Oven-roasted veggies

½ aubergine, chopped
1 courgette, chopped
Juice from ½ lemon
Organic herb salt, to taste
Water, filtered

Preheat the oven to 200°C or 400°F (Mark 6).

Place the aubergine and courgette in an oven-proof dish lined with baking parchment, sprinkle with the herb salt, a little water and the lemon juice, and place in the oven for 20 minutes, or until the veggies are soft.
Stir into your pasta.

Pasta with courgette boats

This is one of my all-time favourite dishes and I am so happy to finally be able to share it.

SERVES: 2

2 large courgettes
2 handfuls of cocktail tomatoes
15 black olives
½ red onion
2 cups of brown rice penne
Dry-roasted cashew nuts (page 55) - optional to scatter on top

Preheat the oven to 200°C or 400°F (Mark 6).

Halve the courgettes and use a pointed spoon to extract the soft centre, leaving a 1 cm-wide surround so that they retain their shape.

Chop the extracted part of the courgette, the cocktail tomatoes, olives and red onion and mix everything in a bowl.

Cover the inside of an oven-proof dish with baking parchment and place the courgette halves on it with the cut sides up.

Spoon the vegetable mix into the courgette 'boats', sprinkle a few drops of water on top and place in the middle of the oven for 25 minutes.

Meanwhile, cook the pasta/rice according to the instructions on the package.

The courgettes are done when a knife easily cuts through them.

Serve with a big salad – this is pure angel food!

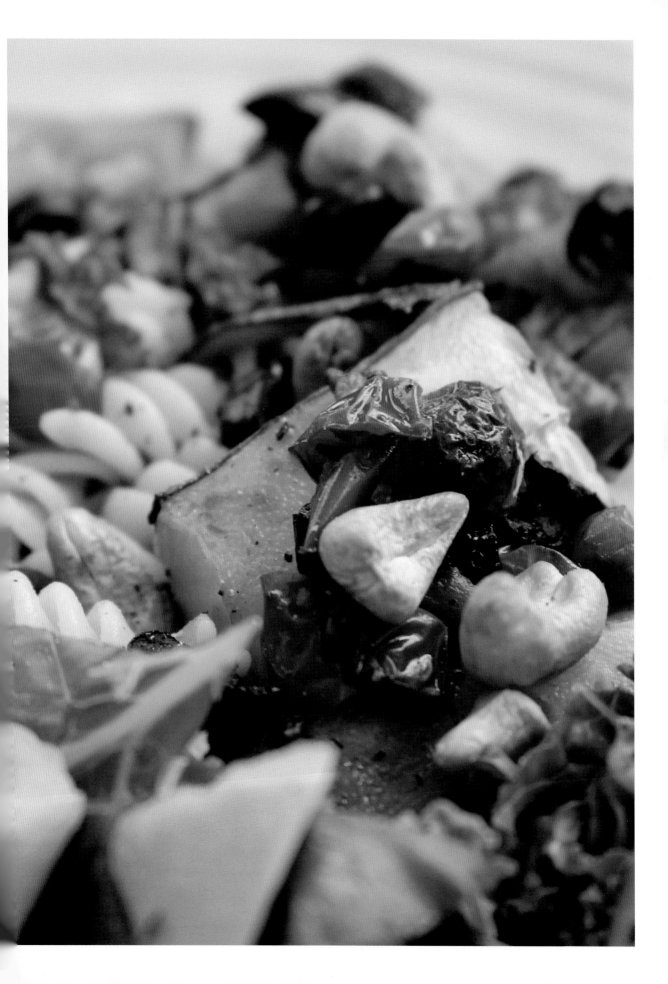

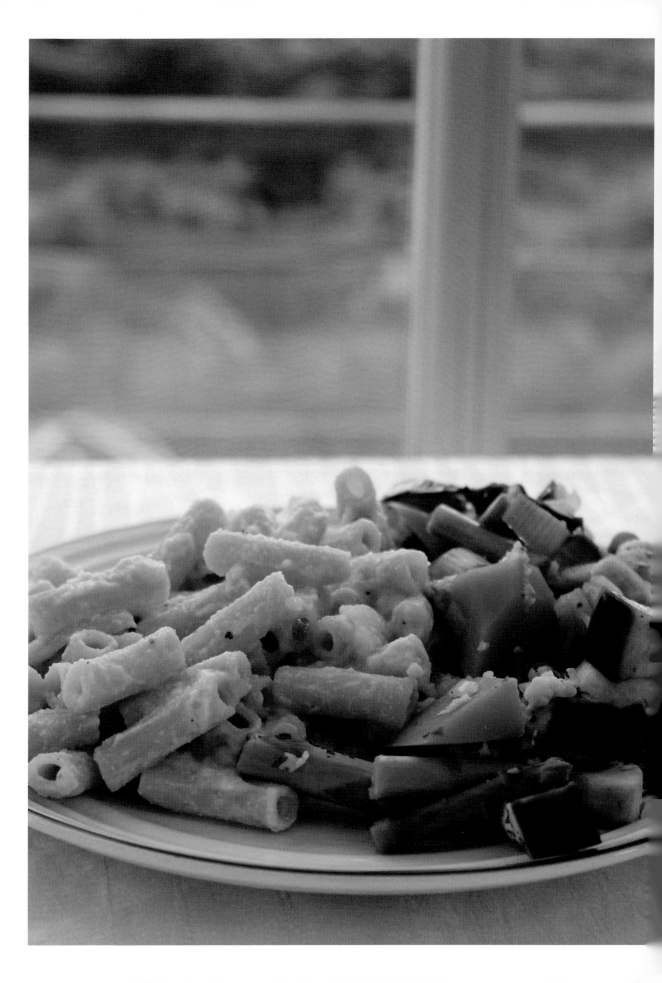

Creamy pasta sauce

I find few foods to be more comforting than pasta with a really creamy sauce, so I am including my two favourite recipes here. This first one is very kind to the system, deliciously creamy and one which I was able to have early on since it doesn't contain any advanced foods, like nuts. It does, however, include gluten-free flour so it is not quite as gentle as a *'Humble and Healing'* recipe.

SERVES: 4

2 shallots, chopped
2 cloves garlic, minced
2 cups of liquid (you can use almond milk **or** oat milk **or** cooking water from the pasta – **or** a mixture of all three)
1 tbsp gluten-free flour
½ cup cold filtered water
4 tbsp nutritional yeast
Black pepper, a few twists
2 tsp lemon juice
Himalayan pink salt or Herbamare, to taste

Serve with:
Gluten-free spaghetti or other pasta

In a ceramic saucepan steam-fry the shallots and garlic in a dash of water until soft. Turn down the heat.

Stir half the liquid into the shallots and bring to a simmer.

Mix the gluten-free flour with the **cold** water and stir until you have a smooth paste.

Add the flour mix and the rest of the liquid into the sauce and stir until it has thickened slightly, then turn off the heat.

Stir in the nutritional yeast, black pepper, lemon juice and season with salt to taste.

Stir into your pasta.

Optional veggie additions to the creamy pasta sauce

Mushrooms — slice and steam-fry briefly in a dash of water and some Tamari sauce in a ceramic saucepan. Stir into the pasta sauce when done.

1 cup of green peas — steam or boil beforehand and stir into the sauce towards the end.

1 large courgette — slice and stir into the sauce towards the end so it retains its crunch. Stir the sauce into your pasta, sprinkle with some fresh chives or basil on top and enjoy.

'Cheesy' cashew cream sauce

This creamy pasta sauce contains cashews and is one of my absolute favourite staple foods in the kitchen. Not only does it work beautifully as a pasta sauce but it can also be used in place of a béchamel sauce in casseroles and it is glorious when mixed in with potatoes for a really creamy mash.

SERVES: 4

1 cup of cashews, soaked overnight in filtered water
½ cup filtered water
A squeeze of lemon juice
$\frac{1}{6}$ cup nutritional yeast
½ tsp onion powder
¼ tsp garlic powder
Organic herb salt or Himalayan pink salt – to taste
Black pepper

Serve with:
Gluten-free spaghetti or other pasta

Drain and rinse the cashews, then blend all the ingredients in a food processor/blender, such as a Nutribullet, until you have a smooth and creamy consistency.

Stir into pasta and add your favourites – you can, for example, choose one or a few of these:

- Chickpeas, stirred into the pasta with the sauce

- Baby spinach – this wilts beautifully into the pasta with a dash of boiling water

- Oven-roasted cocktail tomatoes, scattered on top

- Mushrooms, sliced and cooked with a dash of Tamari sauce

- Olives

- Capers

- Broccoli, steamed but still with a bit of crunch

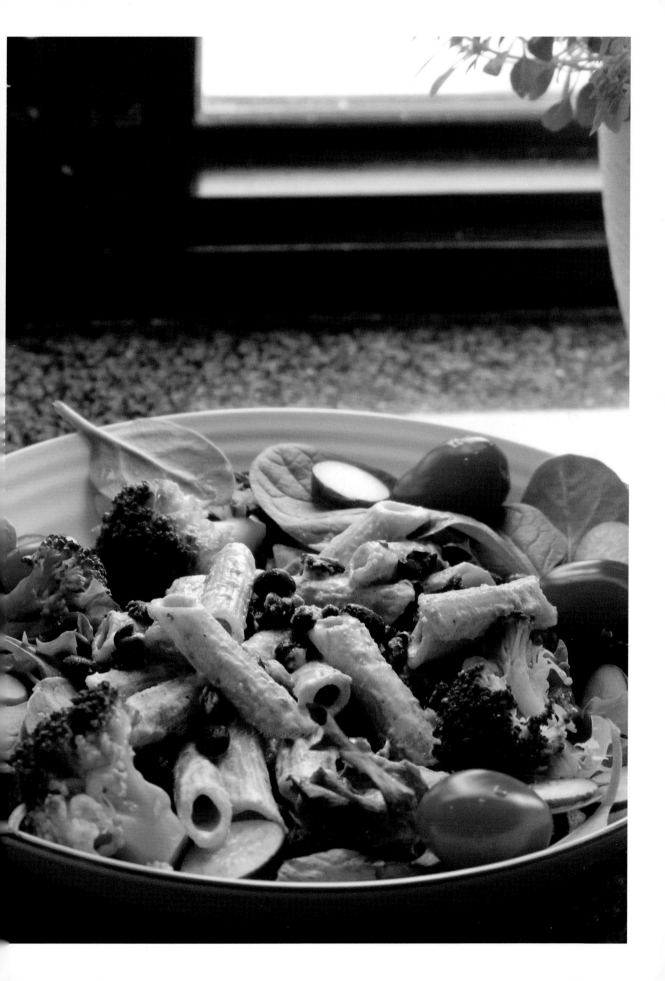

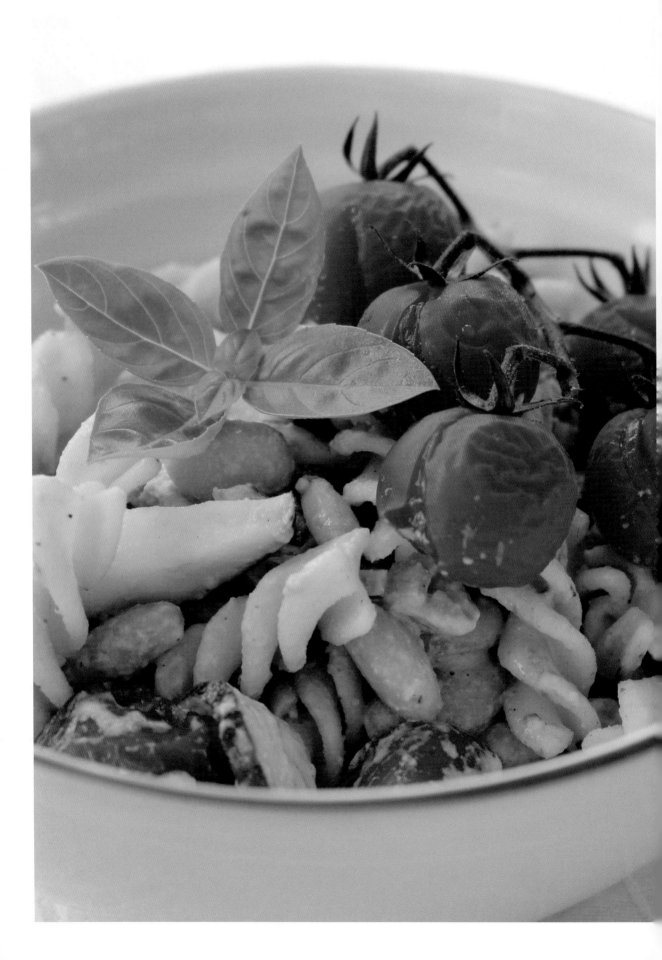

Pesto pasta with cannellini beans

The pesto recipe on the next page is part of this pasta recipe and together they make such a lovely, creamy dish. If you haven't yet tried roasting cocktail tomatoes in the oven, you are in for quite a treat! They are so sweet and yummy and add a perfect, unexpected touch here; just make sure to mix them in carefully at the end as they may break easily.

SERVES: 2-3

½ red onion, chopped
½ lemon
10 cocktail tomatoes
1 clove of garlic, unpeeled
Organic herb salt, to taste
Black pepper
Himalayan pink salt
1 can of cannellini beans or soak ½ cup dried cannellini beans and cook them as per the instructions on the package
3 cups of brown rice fusilli
1 courgette, chopped
Fresh basil leaves

Plus pesto
(see recipe on page 98)

Preheat the oven to 200°C or 400°F (Mark 6).

Place the red onion in a bowl and squeeze the lemon on top. Set aside.

Place the cocktail tomatoes on baking parchment together with the unpeeled clove of garlic.

Grind some salt and pepper over the tomatoes and a sprinkling of water.

Bake in the oven for 25 minutes.

After 15 minutes take out the garlic, peel and place in the blender with the rest of the pesto ingredients, as per the Pesto recipe on page 98.

Cook the pasta according to the instructions on the package.

Rinse the beans in a sieve and drain the hot pasta water over the beans to warm them up.

Mix all the ingredients including the courgette in a big bowl, season to taste and serve with fresh basil on top.

The perfect green pesto

This is a delicious pesto that goes perfectly with a big pasta salad. I love serving it to friends as even those who are not plant-based come back asking for seconds… and thirds! Since the garlic should ideally be roasted in the oven, it is a good idea to cook some oven-roasted vegetables at the same time.

1 clove garlic, unpeeled
¹⁄₃ cup pine nuts
1 full pot of fresh basil leaves
3 tsp lemon juice
Organic herb salt, to taste
Black pepper
½ tsp maple syrup
2 tbsp filtered water

Preheat the oven to 200°C or 400°F (Mark 6).

Place the unpeeled garlic in an oven-proof dish and roast for 10 minutes.

Heat a ceramic frying pan and pour in the pine nuts. Roast in the dry pan on a medium heat until they start getting colour – then immediately take the pan off the heat and set aside.

Tear off the basil leaves and place in a blender.

Pour the lemon juice over the basil and add the rest of the ingredients, including the roasted pine nuts and the water.

Blend until smooth.

Stir into your favourite pasta and veggies.

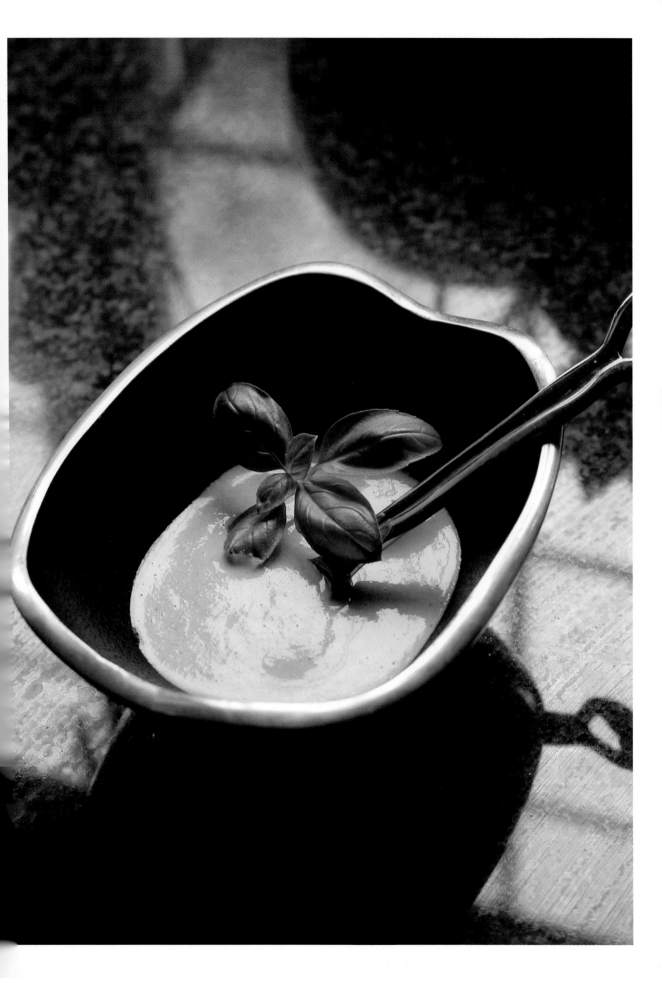

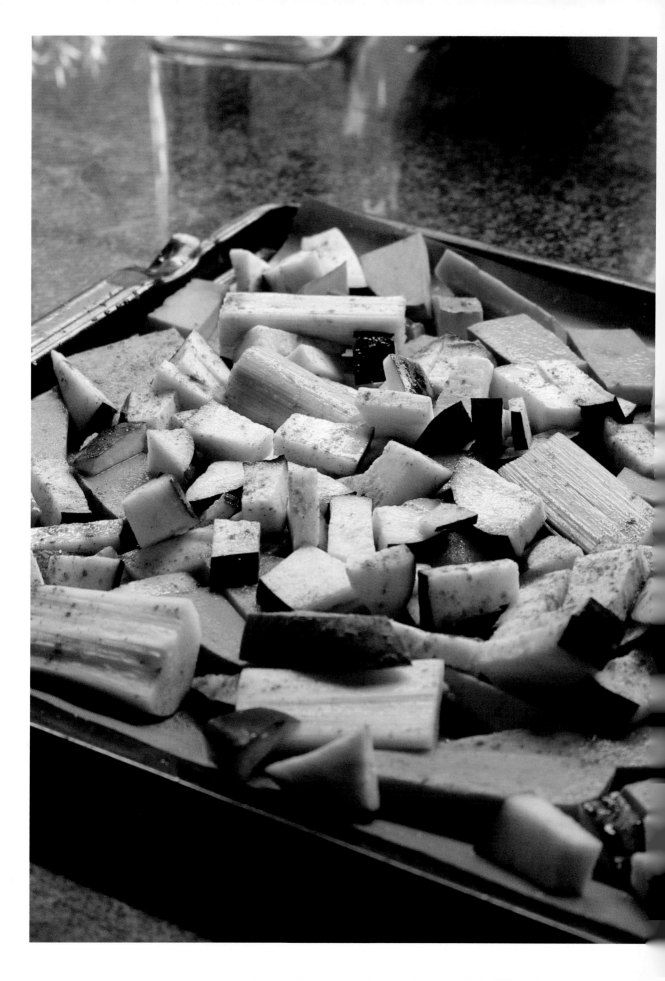

Potatoes

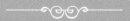

Sweet potato wedges

I like to cook lots in veggies in the oven in one go so whenever I make these sweet potato wedges I take the opportunity to roast, for example aubergine, leek, courgette, parsnips and/ or carrots too. The sweet potato wedges make a perfect side dish as they go with so much, they are also super-tasty the next day and because they don't need to be warmed up they make an excellent snack or addition to a packed lunch.

SERVES: 1

1 large sweet potato, cut into very thin wedges
a) Turmeric and cayenne pepper
or
b) Cinnamon and nutmeg
A wedge of lemon

Preheat the oven to 220°C or 425°F (Mark 7).

Place your sweet potato wedges on some baking parchment on a baking sheet and space them out properly.

Sprinkle either one of the spice combinations on top and add a sprinkling of water.

Place in the oven for 20 minutes or until the wedges are soft and slightly crispy. You can turn the grill function on/put them under your grill for five minutes at the end.

Serve with lemon juice squeezed on top (don't skip that as it makes them just divine!) and a big green salad on the side. Simple yet delicious.

The next two recipes are the perfect way to use up leftover potatoes, and by using different spices you will keep it interesting. Both make lovely side dishes for brunch and are also delicious when served with garlic-infused spinach (page 152).

Sautéed potatoes

Sautéed (or fried) potatoes have always been a favourite of mine so I had to come up with a way of cooking them without oils. You need a good ceramic pan for this, otherwise they will just stick to the bottom – it may take some practice but is worth it in the end as the result is delicious with some nice colour to it.

SERVES: 1

2 large potatoes, boiled, cooled

Seasoning:
¼ tsp paprika powder
¼ tsp onion powder
Himalayan pink salt
Black pepper

Cut the potatoes into ½ cm-thick slices.

Heat a ceramic pan, add a couple of tablespoons of filtered water and wait until it sizzles, then add the potato slices.

Cook on a medium heat; keep adding just a dash of water if the potato slices seem to be sticking to the bottom and use a spatula to move them around. They will soon get some colour; flip them over and repeat.

Add another little splash of water and stir in the seasoning to coat the slices.

Enjoy with your favourite salad, garlic-infused spinach (page 152) or oven-roasted veggies.

Oven-roasted potato chips

SERVES: 1

2 large potatoes, boiled, cooled

Seasoning:
½ tsp cumin and a sprinkling of cayenne pepper
or
1 sprig of fresh rosemary and Himalayan pink salt to taste
or
¼ tsp paprika powder and ¼ tsp onion powder

Set the oven to grill – or if you do not have that function, turn it to 220°C or 425°F (Mark 7) or heat your grill on full.

Cut the potatoes into ½ cm thick slices.

Cover a baking tray with baking paper, spread the potatoes on the paper and sprinkle the seasoning on top with a little filtered water.

Cook in the oven for 10 minutes or until the potatoes are starting to get some colour.

Serve as a snack with a green salad, or as a side dish, or as a main course with a big green salad, if you make loads.

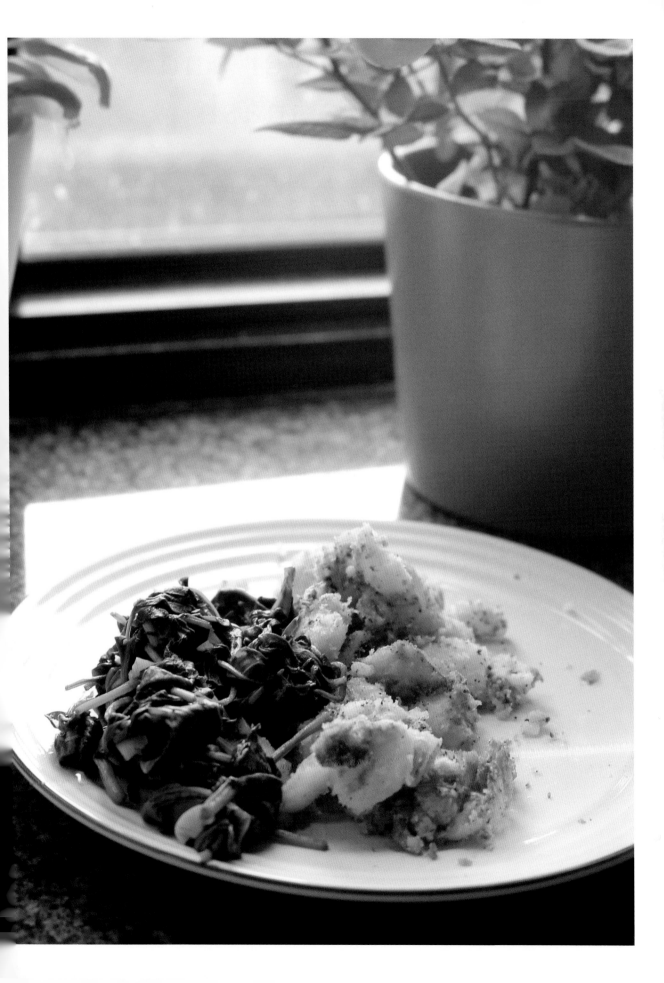

Cauliflower and potato mash

I know that the thought of having just mash as a main course with loads of raw greens may seem a bit unusual but before I was able to have beans and lentils that's how I did it and it worked wonders for me. Do note that organic herb salt is great here as the herbs bring the most delicious flavours to the mash.

SERVES: 2-3
AS A MAIN DISH

4 large potatoes, chopped
½ cauliflower, chopped
1 clove garlic, raw or roasted,
minced – optional
Himalayan pink salt or
Herbamare, to taste

Boil or steam the potatoes and cauliflower separately until soft.

Reserve ½ cup of the boiling water from the potatoes or steamer.

Mash the potatoes and cauliflower together and add as much of the water as you like to get a nice consistency.

Mix in the garlic if you wish to include that, and salt or herb salt until you are happy with the seasoning.

Serve with a big green salad on the side, or have it with, for example, black beans.

Mashed sweet potato

SERVES: 4

3 large sweet potatoes, chopped
1½ cups oat milk
Nutmeg, a sprinkling
Himalayan pink salt, to taste

Boil or steam the sweet potato until soft.

Heat the oat milk in a pot until it is just about to start boiling, stir in the nutmeg and turn off the heat.

Mash the sweet potatoes, add Himalayan pink salt to taste and keep stirring in the oat milk until you are happy with the consistency.

Serve as a main dish with, for example, roasted vegetables, or as a side dish.

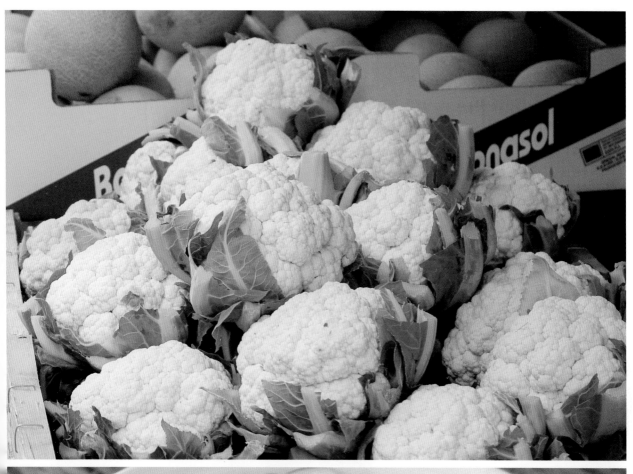

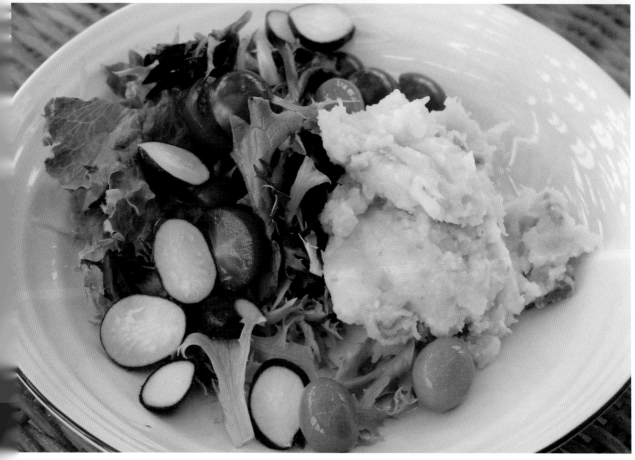

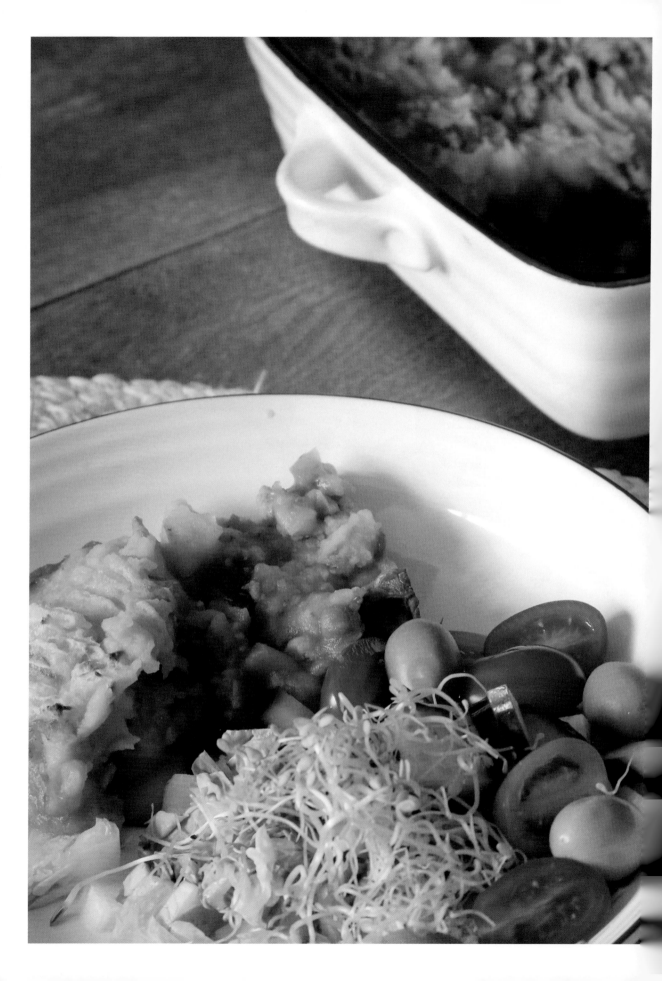

Gardener's pie

The mash:

4 large potatoes, washed and quartered
1 medium-sized sweet potato, washed and quartered into pieces the same size as the potato
Himalayan pink salt, to taste
¾ cup oat milk

The gravy:

1 onion, chopped
2 cloves garlic, minced
8 large mushrooms, sliced
2 tsp Tamari sauce
Black pepper
1 tbsp gluten-free flour
1 cup + ¾ cup cold filtered water
More filtered water, see instructions below

The veggies:

1 can chopped tomatoes
½ cauliflower, cut into very small florets
2 carrots (1 cup), chopped
Water, filtered
1 cup frozen peas
Himalayan pink salt, to taste

Preheat the oven to 180°C or 350°F (Mark 4).

1. The mash

Add the potatoes and sweet potatoes to a pot of boiling water. Cook until they are soft and then drain.

Heat the oat milk in a pan and when it is just about to start boiling, turn off the heat and pour it on top of the potatoes.

Mash and add salt to taste.

2. The gravy

In a ceramic saucepan steam-fry the onion and garlic in a dash of water until soft.

Add the mushrooms to the pan and cook until they have released most of their liquid and start getting some colour.

Add one cup of water, the Tamari sauce and black pepper.

Add the flour to a mug and gradually stir in the cold water; keep stirring until you have a smooth paste, then add this to the mushrooms, stir and bring to the boil.

Allow the gravy to thicken for a couple of minutes, then turn off the heat.

3. The veggies

Put the tomatoes, cauliflower and carrots into a separate pot and add enough water to cover them.

Bring to the boil and cook until the cauliflower starts softening – approximately 10 minutes.

Add the peas and cook for another five minutes.

Add salt to taste.

4. Assembling the gardener's pie:

Pour the tomato, cauliflower and carrot sauce into an oven-proof dish.

Pour the mushroom gravy over the tomato sauce.

Smother with the mashed potatoes on top and ruffle with a fork.

Place the dish in the oven for 20 minutes.

After 20 minutes, place under the grill and allow the mash to get some colour for approximately 10 minutes. Serve with a lovely green salad.

Potato and veggie bake

SERVES: 4

1 onion, chopped
1 clove garlic, pressed
5 large tomatoes, chopped or
1 can chopped tomatoes
1 tsp Tamari sauce
1 tsp organic herb salt
2 tsp oregano or
herbes de Provence
1½ - 2 cups boiled filtered water
3 medium-sized potatoes, cut into thin slices or square strips
1 large courgette, thinly sliced lengthways
1 aubergine, thinly sliced lengthways
1 medium-sized sweet potato, cut into the same shape as the potatoes
1 cup pitted black olives, chopped
½ lemon

Preheat the oven to 200°C or 400°F (Mark 6).

In a ceramic saucepan steam-fry the onion and garlic in a dash of water until soft.

Add the tomatoes, spices and herbs and cook until you have a lovely tomato sauce. It should be quite runny so keep adding water as needed.

Layer an oven-proof dish with potatoes on the bottom, then courgette, aubergine, sweet potato, olives and finally the tomato sauce so that it just about covers everything.

Use a dish with a close-fitting lid and place in the oven.

Cook for approximately 40 minutes, until a knife cuts easily through the vegetables in the centre. *Take the foil off and* place the dish back in the oven for another 10 minutes, to give it some colour on top.

Serve with a green salad and squeeze some lemon on top of everything – lemon and sweet potato is a match made in heaven!

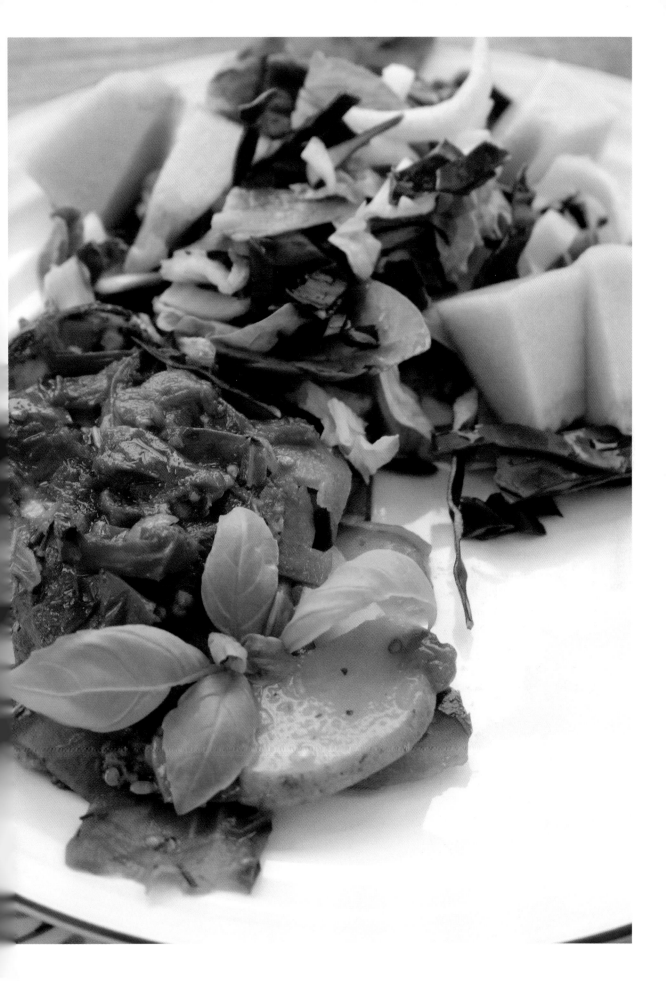

Creamy mashed potatoes with mushroom sauce

SERVES: 4

Mashed potatoes:
10 potatoes, for example King Edward's, peeled and cut into small cubes
½ – 1 cup 'Cheesy' cashew cream sauce (see page 94)
Oat milk – optional

Mushroom sauce:
1 onion, chopped
8 large mushrooms, chopped
2 tsp Tamari sauce
Oat milk
1 tsp dried rosemary
1 bay leaf
Organic herb salt, to taste
Black pepper, to taste
2 tsp gluten-free flour
3 tbsp cold filtered water
1 tsp brown rice miso paste

Serve with:
Boiled or steamed green peas

Mashed potatoes:

Place the potatoes in boiling water and cook until soft.

Pour out the water.

Mash with a potato masher or fork, and bit by bit pour in the cashew cream sauce, mashing well until you are happy with the consistency.

Warm up some oat milk and add to the mash for a looser consistency.

Mushroom sauce:

In a ceramic saucepan steam-fry the onion in a dash of water until soft.

Add the mushrooms and cook until browned. This is easily done by letting the water evaporate quite a lot before pouring a bit more water in to prevent the mushrooms from sticking to the pan.

Stir in the Tamari sauce, oat milk, rosemary, bay leaf, herb salt and black pepper, to taste.

Mix the flour with the cold water until you have a smooth paste.

Once the sauce is simmering on a medium heat, slowly stir in the flour-mix and allow the sauce to thicken. Add more oat milk if you want a looser consistency.

Finally, turn off the heat and stir in the miso paste – do not allow to boil.

Add the mash to four plates and spoon the mushroom sauce on top.

Serve with green peas and a green salad.

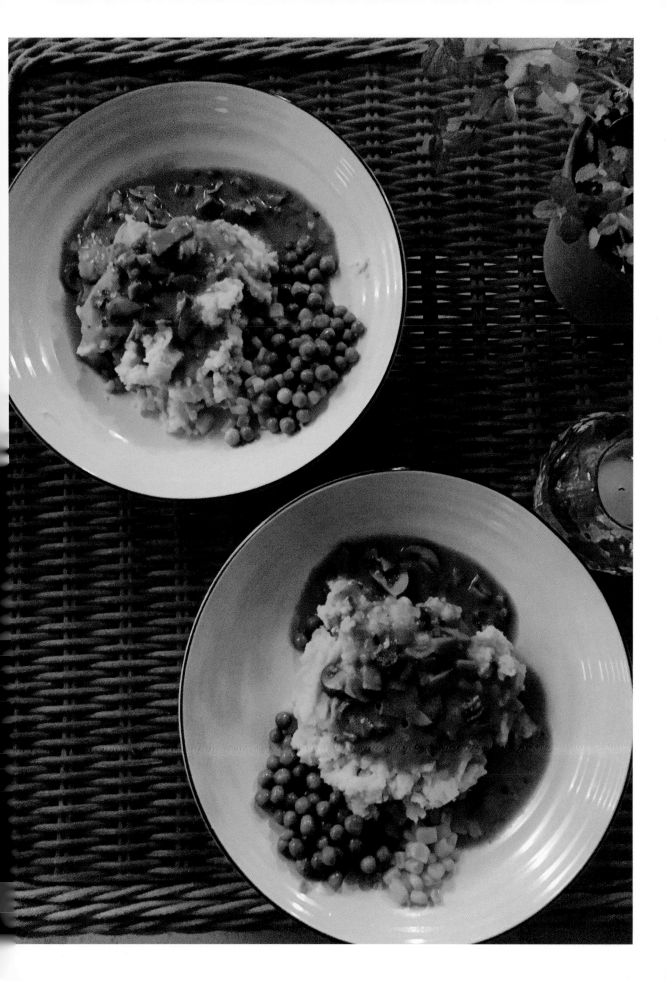

Beans

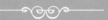

Black bean and sweet potato stew

SERVES: 2

½ onion, chopped
½ leek, sliced
1 cup mushrooms, sliced
½ sweet potato, chopped
Tamari sauce
Cayenne pepper
Organic herb salt
Oregano
1 can organic black beans,
rinsed, or ½ cup black beans,
soaked overnight and cooked as
per the instructions on
the package

Serve with:
1 cup Basmati rice
or potatoes
Fresh coriander

Steam-fry the onion in a ceramic saucepan with a dash of water for two minutes.

Stir in the leek, mushrooms, sweet potato and seasonings and cook until the sweet potatoes are soft.

Add the beans and turn the heat to very low. Do not allow to boil but keep warm for five minutes.

Serve with brown Basmati rice or potatoes, fresh coriander and a huge green salad.

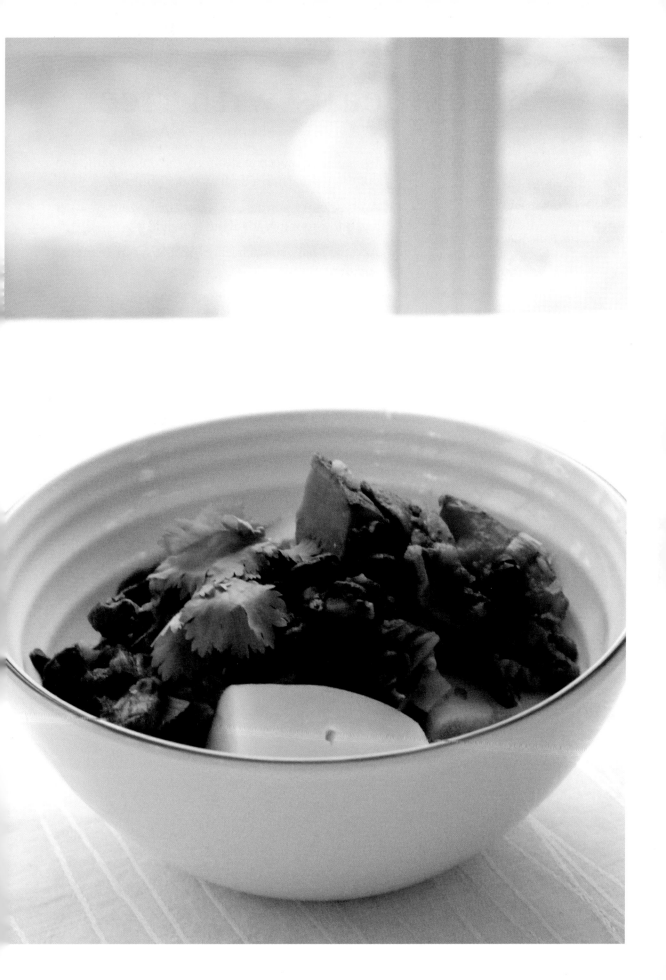

Black beans with rice

SERVES: 2

1 onion, chopped
1 clove garlic, minced
1 cup butternut squash, chopped
into small pieces
1 tsp curry powder
1 can organic black beans,
rinsed, or ½ cup black beans,
soaked overnight and cooked
as per the instructions on the
package
1 handful fresh spinach
Himalayan pink salt, to taste
Black pepper, a few twists
¼ tsp maple syrup
½ tsp Tamari sauce
Water, filtered, for cooking

Serve with:
½ cup Basmati rice
Fresh coriander

In a ceramic saucepan steam-fry the onion, garlic and butternut squash in a dash of water until soft.

Add the curry powder and a few tablespoons of water and allow to infuse for about a minute.

Add the beans, spinach leaves, maple syrup, seasoning and Tamari sauce.

Warm it all up but do not bring to the boil, in order to retain all the nutrients.

Check seasoning and add salt if you wish.

Serve with Basmati rice, fresh coriander, a green salad and perhaps sauerkraut on the side.

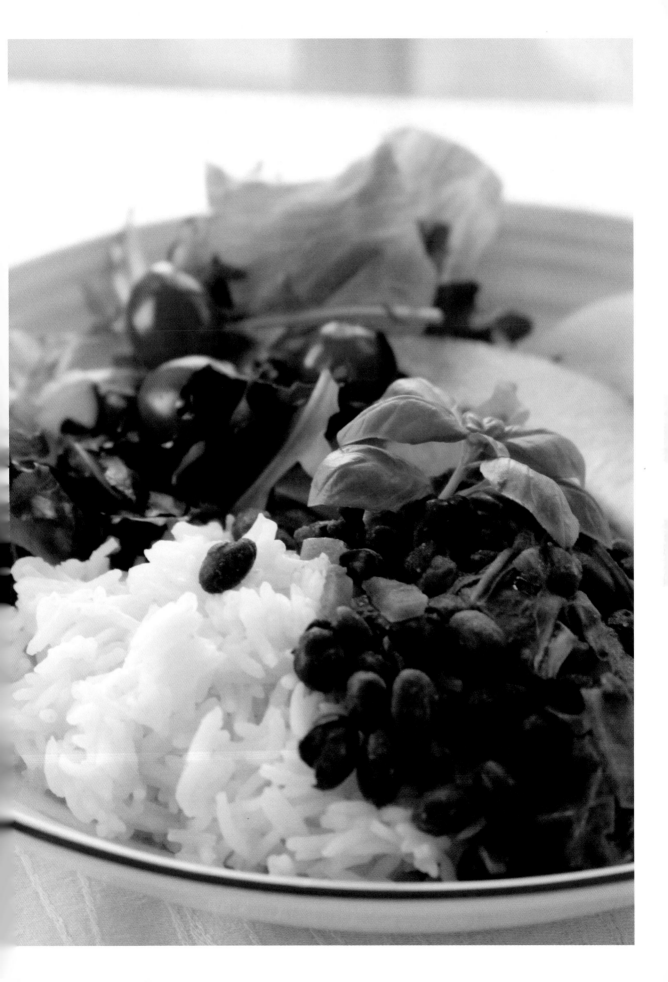

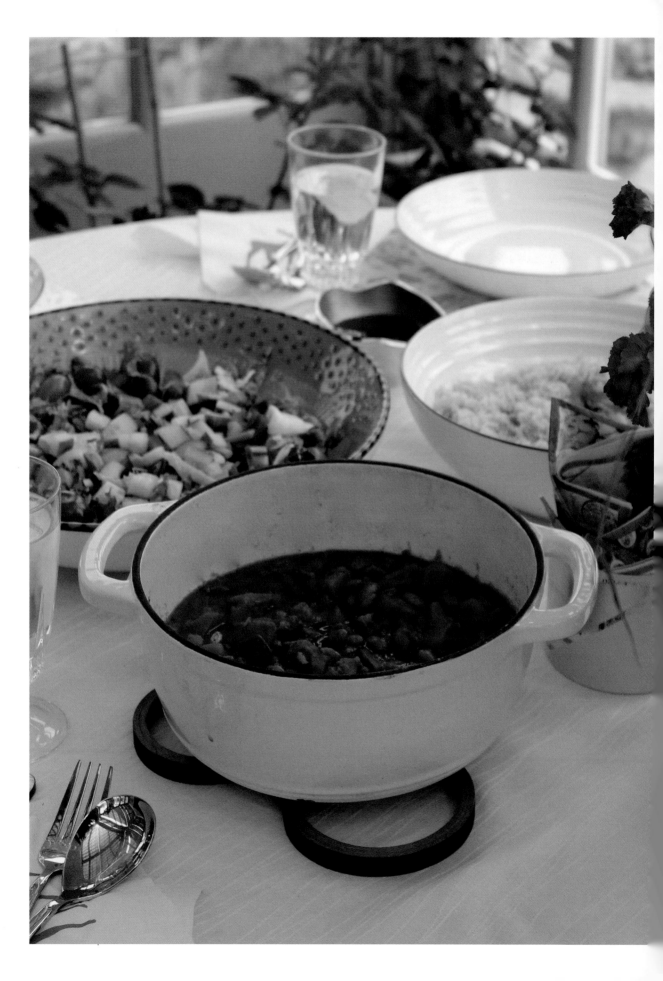

Adzuki bean chilli

SERVES: 4

*³/₄ cup adzuki beans – soaked
overnight, rinsed and drained
1 yellow onion, chopped
2 cloves garlic, pressed
½ butternut squash, chopped
1 stalk celery, chopped
½ fresh red chilli pepper,
finely chopped
Any leftover veggies
from making vegetable broth
(see page 136) – optional
1 tsp cinnamon
¼ tsp nutmeg
½ tsp mustard seeds
3 tsp fresh ginger, chopped
3 large tomatoes, chopped
3 tsp Tamari sauce
1½ tsp organic herb salt
Black pepper
Fresh coriander – stalks and
leaves separated, stalks chopped
3 cups filtered water*

Serve with:
1½ cups Basmati rice

Place the soaked and rinsed adzuki beans in a pot with 1 litre of filtered water and bring to the boil.

Boil vigorously for 10 minutes; then turn down the heat to medium.

Meanwhile, add a little water to a ceramic saucepan and cook the onion, garlic, butternut squash, celery and chilli on a medium heat for 10 minutes. Keep adding water as needed.

If you are using the leftover veggies from making vegetable broth, this is the time to add those.

Stir in the cinnamon, nutmeg, mustard seeds and ginger and cook for one minute.

Add the tomatoes and some more water and cook for another minute.

Pour the mixture in with the beans, add the Tamari sauce, organic herb salt, as much black pepper as you wish, and mix well.

Add the coriander stalks and let it all cook together until the beans are soft, often another 20-30 minutes.

While the beans are cooking away, cook the rice according to the instructions on the packet.

Check the seasoning of the beans towards the end.

Serve on top of Basmati rice with the coriander leaves scattered on top, a big green salad and some sauerkraut or kimchi on the side.

Pinto bean chilli

This is such a delicious chilli; just remember to place your pinto beans soaking in cold water overnight. I often make this dish when I have people round and just add more vegetables to make a bigger batch.

SERVES: 2-3

1 cup pinto beans, soaked overnight
1 onion, chopped
2 cloves garlic, minced
½ leek, sliced thinly
2 carrots, chopped
1 tsp cumin
½ tsp hot paprika powder
2 small fresh red chillies, chopped
¼ tsp cinnamon
1/8 tsp nutmeg
1 tsp maple syrup
1 tsp oregano
3 tsp Tamari sauce
1 tsp Himalayan pink salt
3 cups water, filtered and boiled
2 cups sweet potato, cubed

Serve with:
1½ cups Basmati rice
Fresh coriander
Coconut yoghurt – optional

Rinse the soaked pinto beans and set aside.

In a ceramic saucepan steam-fry the onion, garlic, leek and carrots in a dash of water until soft. Keep adding water as needed.

Add all the seasonings, stir well so that everything is evenly coated and allow to cook for a few minutes before you add the water and bring to the boil.

Boil briskly for 10 minutes, then turn down the heat to a simmer.

Cook for at least one hour, adding the sweet potatoes after 30 minutes so as not to overcook them.

While the beans are cooking away, cook the rice according to the instructions on the packet.

The beans can cook for longer to allow the flavours to really infuse – simmering for two hours makes it just fantastic. Do check seasoning before serving as the beans soak it all up and might need more Tamari sauce, for example.

Serve on top of the rice, with coriander and a green salad on the side.

A dollop of coconut yoghurt takes this dish to a whole new level – so delicious!

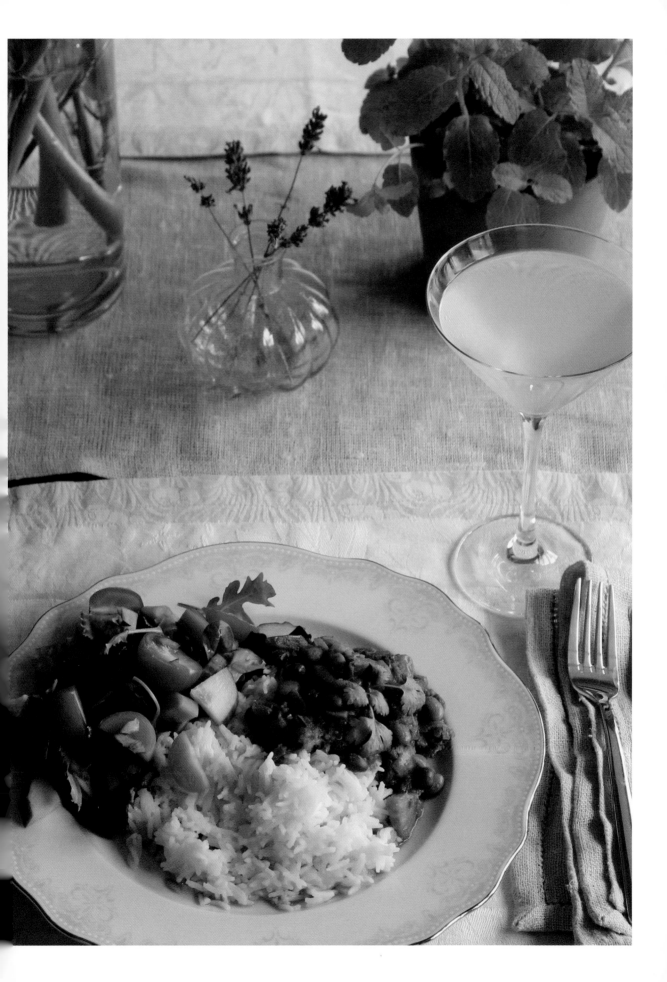

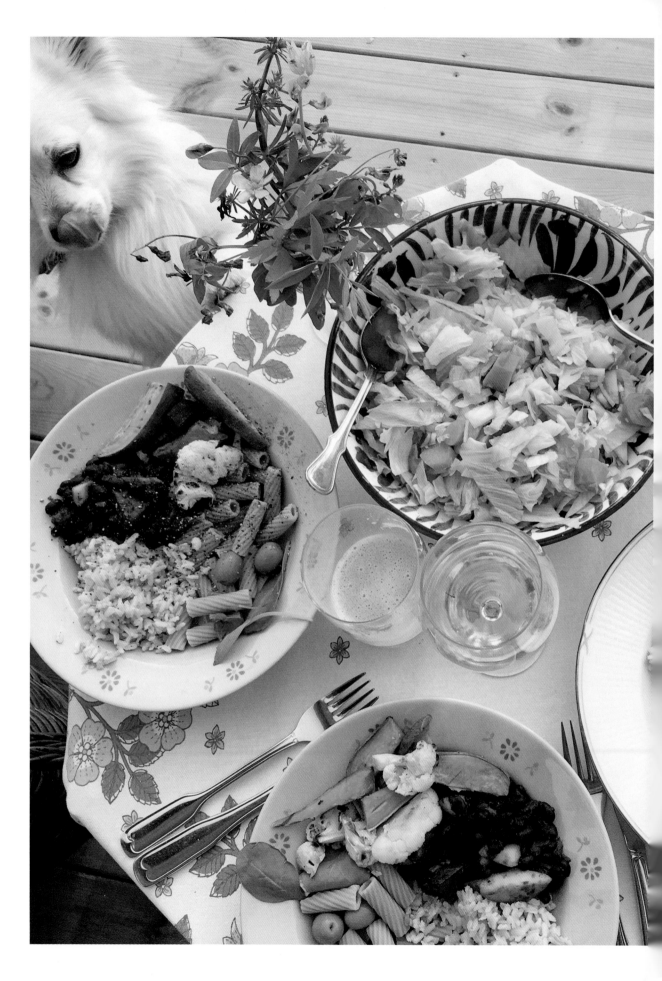

Chilli con todo

SERVES: 2-3

1 onion, chopped
1 clove garlic, minced
3 large tomatoes, chopped
1 cup filtered water
¼ tsp cayenne pepper
A dash of dried chilli pepper
2½ tsp Tamari sauce
1 tsp oregano
A dusting of nutmeg
½ tsp cinnamon
Black pepper
Juice from ½ lemon
1 cup quinoa, cooked
1 can organic black beans,
rinsed, or ½ cup black beans,
soaked overnight and cooked
as per the instructions on the
package

Serve with:
1 cup Basmati rice
Fresh coriander

In a ceramic saucepan, steam-fry the onion and garlic in a dash of water until soft.

Stir in the chopped tomatoes, water, spices and a squeeze of lemon.

Mix in the quinoa and stir. Check the flavour.

Bring the heat down, stir in the black beans and warm up but do not boil.

Serve with the rice, fresh coriander scattered on top and a big green salad.

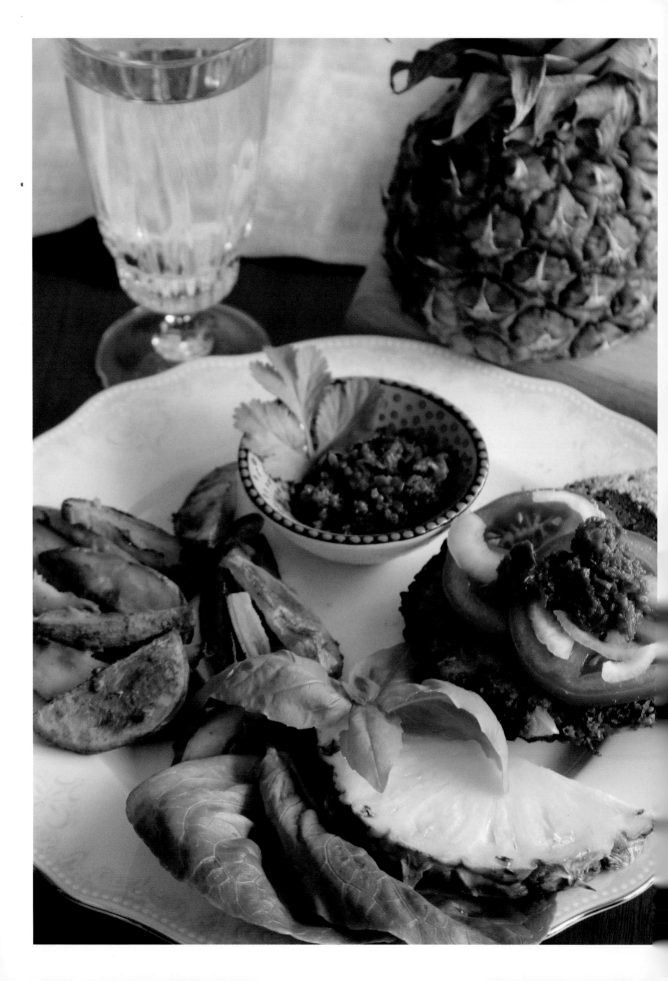

Black bean burgers

Cumin gives these burgers an exotic touch and the paprika adds a lovely kick. The apple sauce and oats help bind the burgers and are super-tasty in the mix.

MAKES 4 BURGERS

2 tsp finely chopped onion
1 can organic black beans, rinsed, or ½ cup black beans, soaked overnight and cooked as per the instructions on the package
½ tsp garlic powder
¼ tsp cumin
¼ tsp hot paprika
¾ tsp organic herb salt or Pink Himalayan salt
⅛ tsp turmeric
1 tbsp finely grated courgette
⅛ cup oats
1 tbsp apple sauce (see page 50)
1 tsp oat milk
Black pepper

Preheat the oven to 220°C or 425°F (Mark 7).

In a ceramic saucepan steam-fry the onion in a dash of water until soft.

Rinse the black beans and pour into a bowl. Mash them up with a fork roughly, so that a few larger beans remain.

In a separate bowl, mix all the spices.

Add the rest of the ingredients, including the spices, to the beans and mix well.

Divide into four equal portions; place each on baking parchment on an oven-proof tray, shaping them first into a ball and then pressing down on them to create four round patties.

Cook in the oven for approximately 20 minutes. For the last five minutes change the setting to grill or fan, or move the tray to your grill, to allow the burgers to get some colour.

Remove from the oven or grill and allow to sit for five minutes as they will firm up slightly. Serve and enjoy.

As a lovely treat I can also recommend having the burgers with the chocolate shake (page 179).

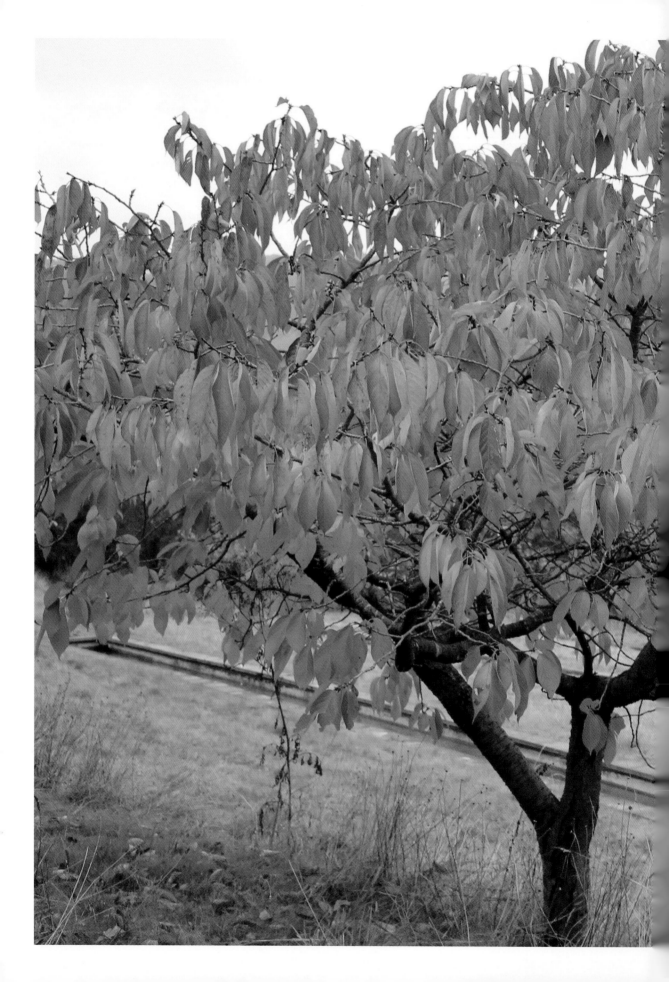

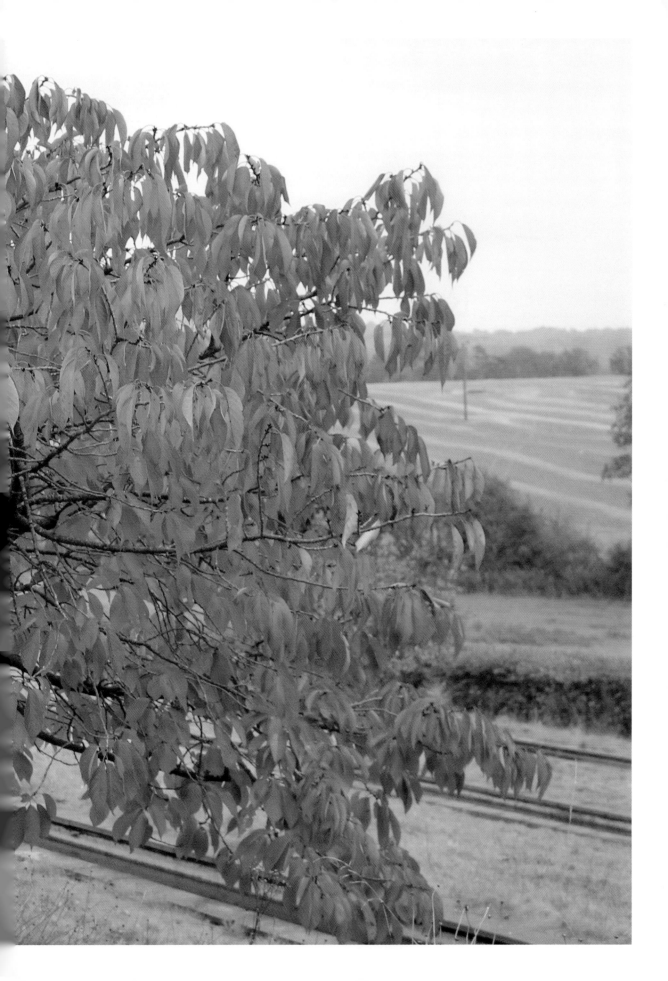

Curries, lentils and soups

Red lentil stew

SERVES: 4

2 cloves garlic, minced
1 yellow onion, chopped
1 tsp cumin
½ tsp paprika
¼ tsp chilli powder
1½ tsp organic herb salt or
Himalayan pink salt
½ leek, sliced thinly across
1 carrot, chopped
2 cups butternut squash,
chopped
1 cup red lentils
4-5 cups filtered water
1 handful spinach

Serve with:
1½ cups brown Basmati rice

In a ceramic saucepan, steam-fry the garlic and onion in a dash of water until soft.

Add the cumin, paprika, chilli and salt, cook for one minute and keep adding water as necessary.

Stir in the leek, carrot and butternut squash, add more water if needed and cook for one minute.

Pour in the lentils and the water so that everything is covered.

Simmer on a low heat until the lentils and butternut squash are soft.

Finally, add the spinach, stir for 30 seconds until it has wilted, and serve right away with the brown rice and a green salad.

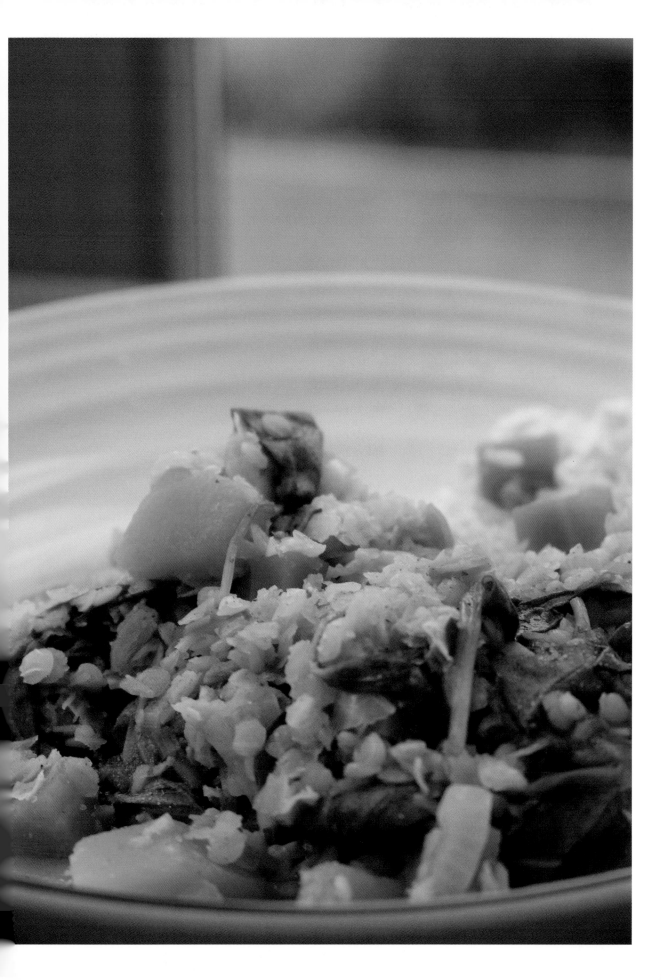

Sweet and easy yellow split-pea stew

I made this on a chilly autumn day when a friend came over for lunch. She has three children and I wanted to give her some inspiration for a quick and simple weekday dish for the family. We realised that you need to make a great big batch of it, as it is such delicious soul food that you will want to go for seconds, and maybe even thirds.

SERVES: 2

1 small yellow onion, chopped
¼ tsp fresh or ground ginger
1 cup yellow split peas
¼ tsp turmeric
5 cups cold water
1 cup sweet potato, cut into chunks
¼ tsp organic herb salt
¼ tsp Himalayan pink salt
2 tsp miso paste

In a ceramic saucepan, steam-fry the onion in a dash of water until soft.

Stir in the ginger and another dash of water to prevent the ingredients from sticking to the bottom.

Add the rest of the ingredients, except the miso paste, bring to the boil, then turn down the heat and simmer until the peas and sweet potato are soft, usually around 40 minutes.

If you think the stew is too watery, you can just turn up the heat for a few minutes and let any excess water evaporate.

Stir in the miso paste and turn off the heat, to help it retain its wonderful health properties.

Enjoy with a big green salad on the side.

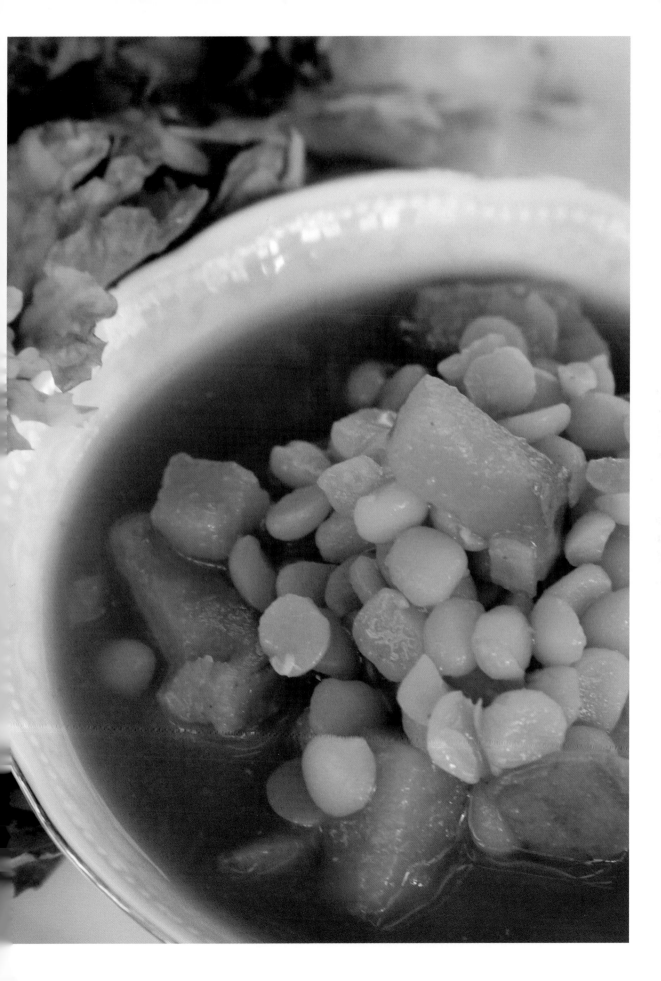

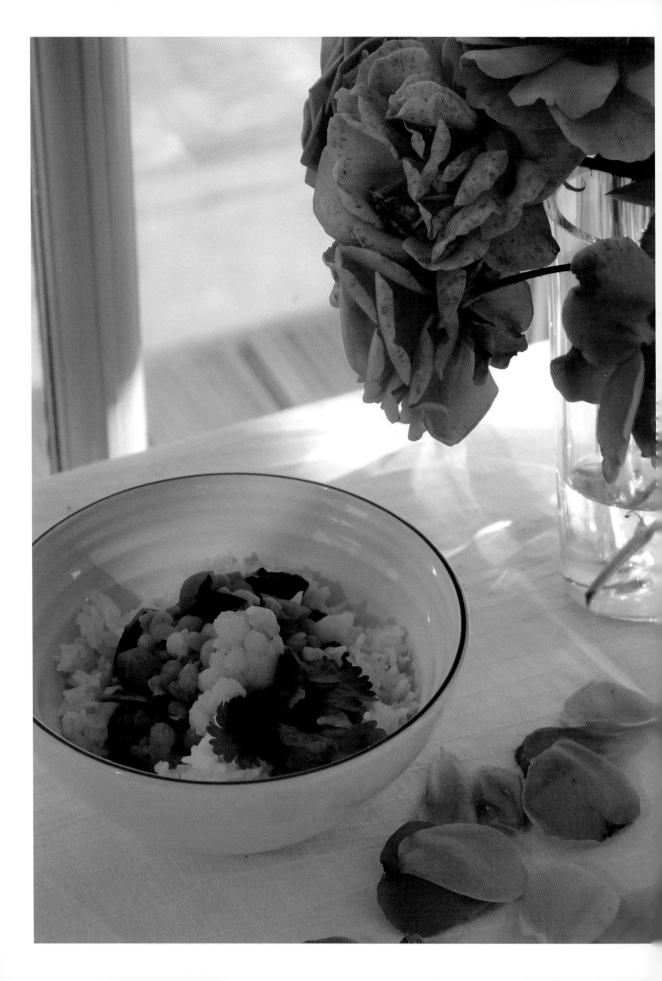

Yellow split-pea and cauliflower stew

This is a delicious and humble dish where all the veggies come together particularly beautifully. The best way to preserve the nutrients in the cauliflower is to steam it, but to save pots and pans you can just let it simmer in the stew until soft – approximately 10 minutes.

SERVES: 4

1 cup yellow split peas
1 tsp turmeric
1 onion, chopped
1 clove garlic, pressed
1 carrot, chopped
1 tsp curry powder
1 tsp fresh ginger, chopped
¼ tsp nutmeg, freshly grated
½ cauliflower, cut into
small florets
2 handfuls spinach
3 ½ cups filtered water
Fresh coriander

Serve with:
1½ cup brown Basmati rice

Bring the yellow split peas to the boil in the water and add the turmeric. Boil on medium heat for 10 minutes.

In a separate pan, steam-fry the onion and garlic in a dash of water until soft.

Add the carrot, curry powder, ginger, grated nutmeg and some more water to the onions; stir well.

Pour in the yellow split peas and the water, and simmer for about 20 minutes:

Version 1:

If you are cooking the cauliflower in the stew, now is the time to add it and simmer for another 10 minutes. Stir in the spinach and watch it wilt beautifully just before serving.

Version 2:

If you choose to steam the cauliflower, do that separately and just stir it into the stew together with the spinach once the stew is done.

Serve with the fresh coriander, rice and a green salad.

Green lentil and pineapple stew

Lentils contain an abundance of vitamins and minerals and bring a goodly amount of protein to the table also. They also take on flavours from spices beautifully so they are perfect in stews and soups. The high protein content makes lentils a more advanced food if you have rheumatoid arthritis and I always have them with a big bowl of leafy green vegetables that help break it all down in the gut.

SERVES: 4

1 cup green lentils, rinsed and soaked overnight if required
5 cups filtered water
1 onion, chopped
2 shallots, chopped finely
½ tsp turmeric powder
1 tsp curry powder
1 tsp paprika powder
½ tsp chilli powder
1 tsp ground ginger
3 tsp organic herb salt or Himalayan pink salt, to taste
1 tsp lemon juice
1 courgette, chopped
2 cups fresh pineapple, chopped
½ cup frozen green peas

Serve with:
1½ cups brown Basmati rice

Cook the green lentils in 4 cups of the filtered water for 10 minutes.

In a saucepan, steam-fry the onion and shallots in a dash of water until soft.

Stir in the spices and the rest of the water, and then bring to the boil.

Stir in the lentils and the rest of the ingredients apart from the peas, bring to the boil, then reduce the heat.

Simmer until the lentils are soft, stirring occasionally.

Add the peas and cook for another five minutes.

Serve with the rice and a big green salad.

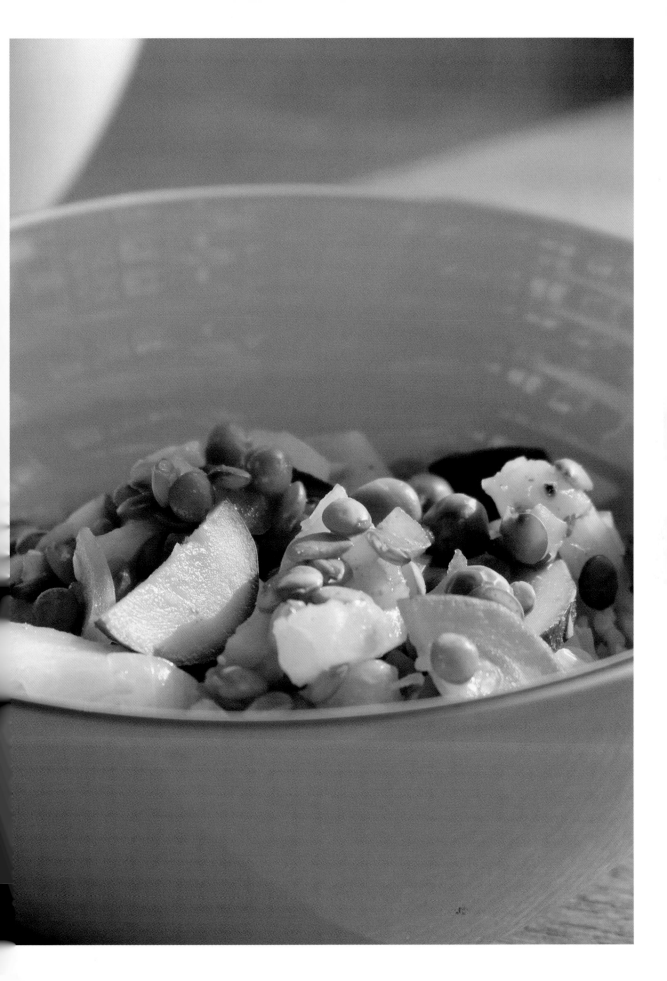

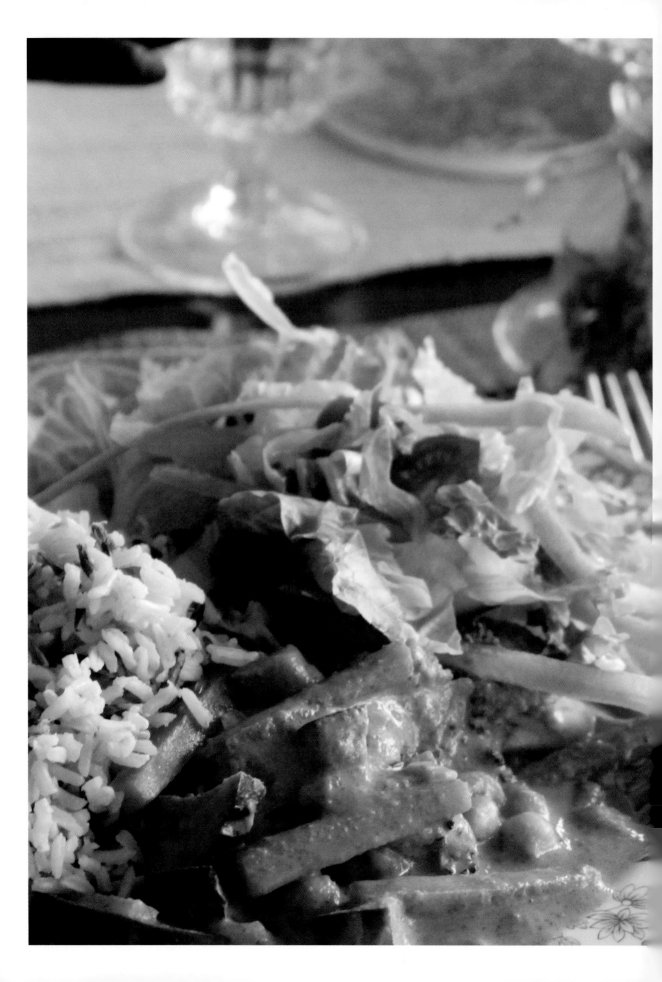

Coconut red curry

This is one of my favourite dishes to make when I have friends over, as it is so quick to prepare and tastes insanely delicious. Chopping the veggies is what takes time; after that, it cooks in about 15 minutes. I always use ready-blended Thai red curry paste, and make sure I get one with no artificial colours, flavourings or preservatives that is suitable for vegans.

SERVES: 2-3

1 yellow onion, sliced into thin half-moons
2 shallots, chopped finely
1 clove garlic, minced
3 tbsp Thai red curry paste (use more for a hotter curry)
1 can coconut milk
1 aubergine, chopped into rectangular pieces
2 carrots, chopped into thin strips
1 broccoli head, chopped into florets
A bunch of fresh coriander, leaves picked off and stems chopped finely
1 lime, cut into four wedges

Serve with:
1½ cups brown Basmati rice

In a saucepan, steam-fry the onions and shallots in a dash of water until soft.

Add the garlic and ginger and cook for a few seconds.

Add the curry paste and 2 tbsp of the coconut milk, stir well and allow the flavours to be released.

Add the rest of the vegetables and stir well.

Pour in the rest of the coconut milk and add the coriander stalks.

Cook on medium/low heat for about 15 minutes or until you are happy with the softness of the vegetables.

Serve with the rice, the coriander leaves scattered on top and a big green salad on the side.

Squeeze the lime juice over it all.

Vegetable broth

I make this vegetable broth on a regular basis as it is perfect to use instead of oils in stir-fries, sauces etc. You can make a big batch to freeze in ice cube trays.

2 large yellow onions, diced
3 cloves of garlic, minced
2 carrots, diced
2 stalks of celery, chopped
1 leek, sliced
2 tomatoes, diced
¼ of a turnip, chopped
1.5 litre cold water
1 bay leaf
A handful of fresh oregano,
coriander and/or thyme
1 tsp herbamare
Himalayan pink salt
1 tbsp Tamari sauce

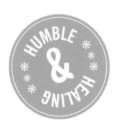

Heat a dash of water in a pot and add the onion, garlic, carrots and celery.

Cook on a medium heat until the vegetables are soft – keep adding water as needed.

Add the rest of the ingredients, except the Tamari sauce, together with the cold water and slowly bring to the boil. By slowly heating everything you will extract the greatest amount of flavour from your veggies.

Once boiling, bring the heat down and let it simmer for an hour.

Towards the end, add Tamari sauce until you are happy with the seasoning; then remove from the heat and allow to cool.

Strain through a fine sieve – the leftover veggies can be used in a soup, or for example in the Adzuki bean chilli (page 117).

Once cooled down the broth can be poured into containers – for example, into ice cube trays to be kept in the freezer and used as needed.

Brown rice miso soup

By adding the unpasteurised miso to hot but not boiling water, the living enzymes are preserved.

½ sheet sushi Nori, torn into
small bits
Fresh spring onion,
a few thin slices
1 cup hot water, not boiling
1 tbsp unpasteurised
brown rice miso

Add the Nori and spring onion to a cup or small bowl, then pour in the water and finally stir in the miso.
Enjoy with for example your homemade sushi (page 64) as a very humble and healing dish.

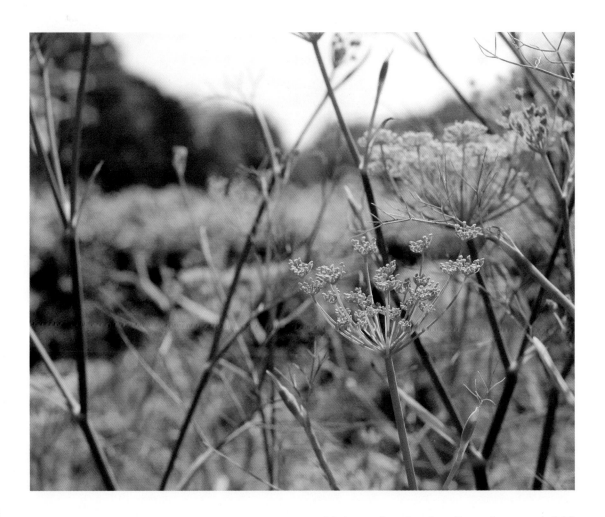

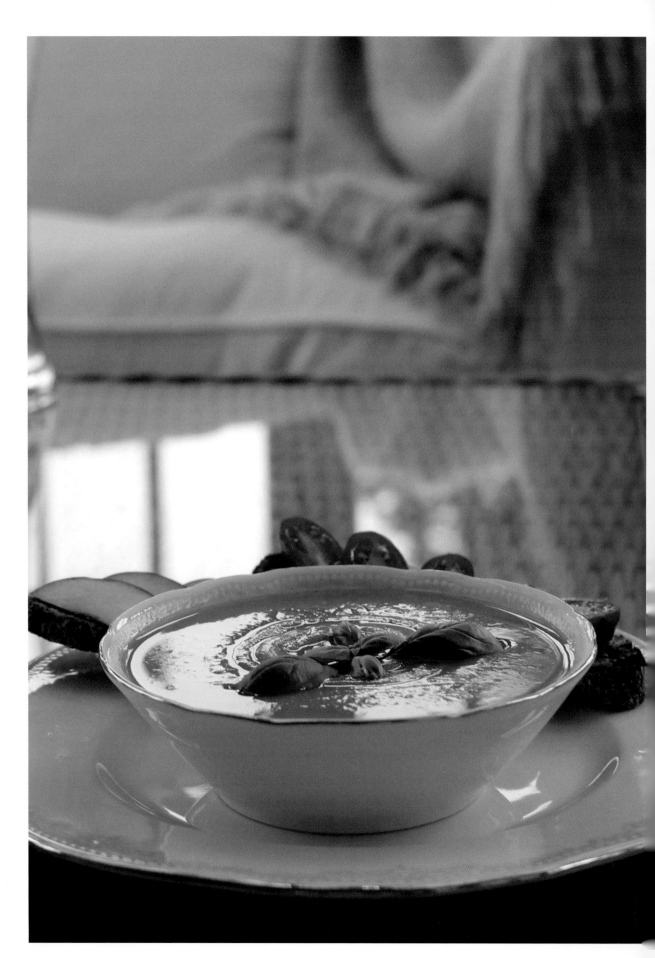

Warming sweet potato and butternut squash soup

SERVES: 4

½ butternut squash, diced
1 large sweet potato, diced
1 small onion, chopped
2 cloves garlic, minced
1 stem of celery, chopped
Leftover vegetables from
the broth recipe (page 136)
– optional
Tamari sauce
Cinnamon
Nutmeg
½ lime
Water, filtered

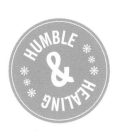

Steam the butternut squash and sweet potato until soft.

Place the onion, garlic and celery in some boiling water and cook for 10 minutes.

If you have leftover veggies from making the veggie broth you can add them now and let them cook together with the above.

Add the Tamari sauce, cinnamon and nutmeg to the boiling water.

In a blender, blend everything until you have a smooth soup. You may need to do this in batches depending on the size of the blender. Check seasoning and bring back to the pot to be heated up again slowly.

Serve with a big green salad.

Try squeezing some lime on top – this gives the soup a wonderful, refreshing flavour.

Yellow split-pea soup

I remember Mum making this for us back in Sweden when I was little and it was one of my favourite foods. It was always so exciting for us kids to see when she put the peas in to soak the night before, as we knew what would be coming the next day.

SERVES: 3-4

1½ cups yellow split peas
6 cups filtered water
½ tsp Himalayan pink salt

Follow the instructions on the packet if the peas need soaking overnight.

Bring the yellow split peas, salt and water to the boil and allow to cook on a low heat for an hour. Stir occasionally and make sure that it doesn't stick to the bottom of the pan.

Check seasoning.

Serve and enjoy with a big green salad on the side.

Finnish summer soup

SERVES: 5-6

Fresh dill, stems and tops separated
Fresh chives, chopped
1 yellow onion
5 large potatoes
4 large carrots
1 cauliflower
6 cups of cold filtered water - or just enough to cover the vegetables
1½ teaspoons Himalayan pink salt
1 tablespoon gluten-free flour
1 ½ cups almond milk
1 cup of frozen peas

Set aside the dill tops and the chives

Chop the onion

Scrub the potatoes and cut into large chunks.

Scrub the carrots and cut into thick slices.

Cut the cauliflower into florets.

Place all the vegetables except the peas in a large pot with the water, salt and dill stems and bring to the boil. Reduce the heat and simmer for 15 minutes

In a mug, stir ½ cup of the almond milk into the flour, mixing well to break up any lumps.

Add the peas to the simmering vegetables, pour in the rest of the almond milk and stir in the flour mixture.

Simmer for a couple of minutes, stirring occasionally.

Turn off the heat and sprinkle the dill and chives over before serving.

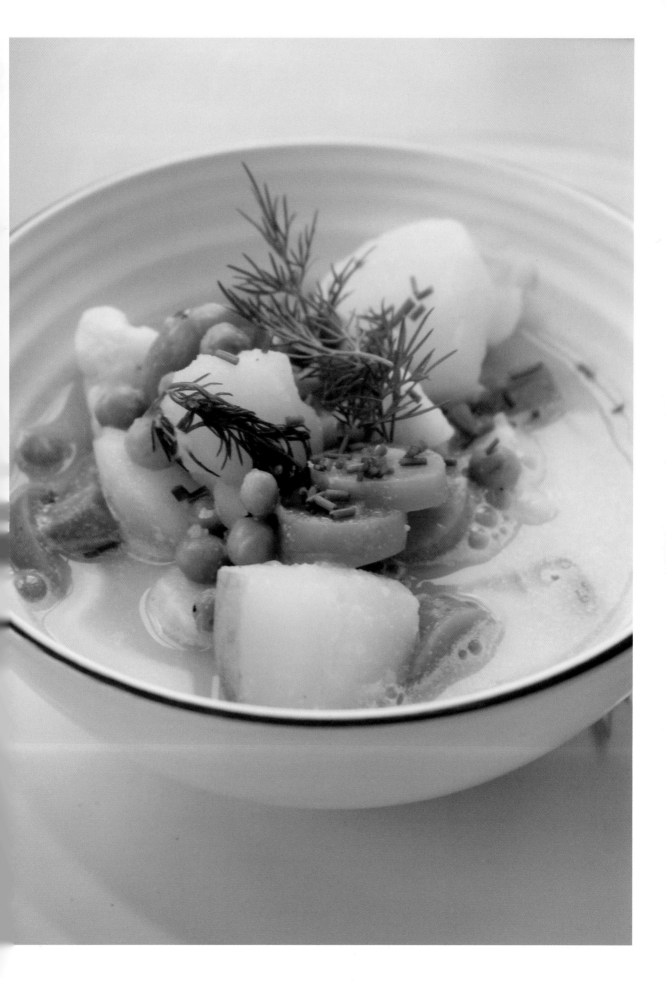

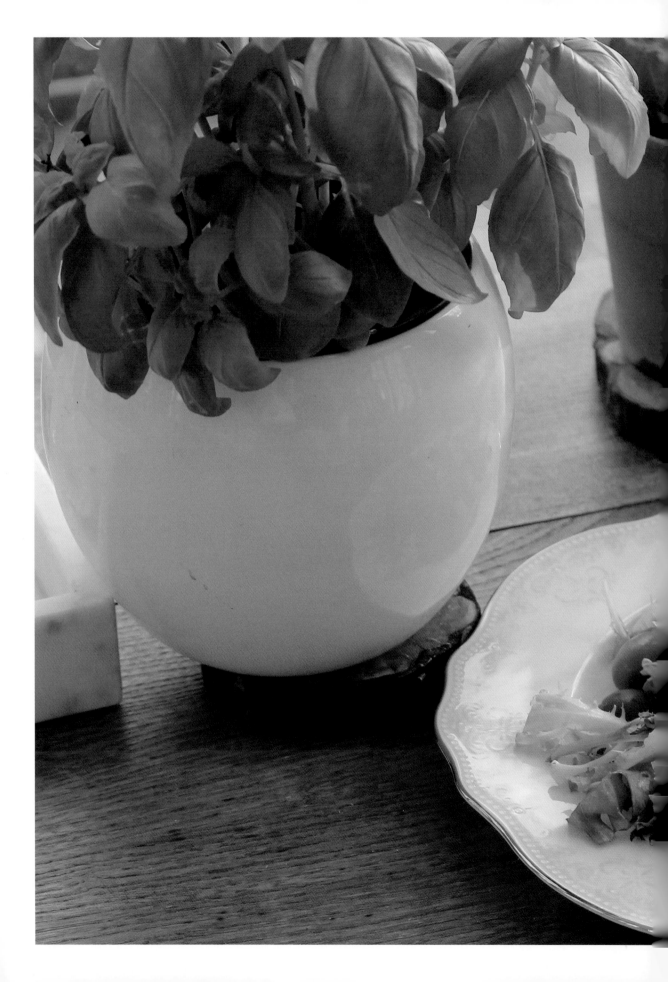

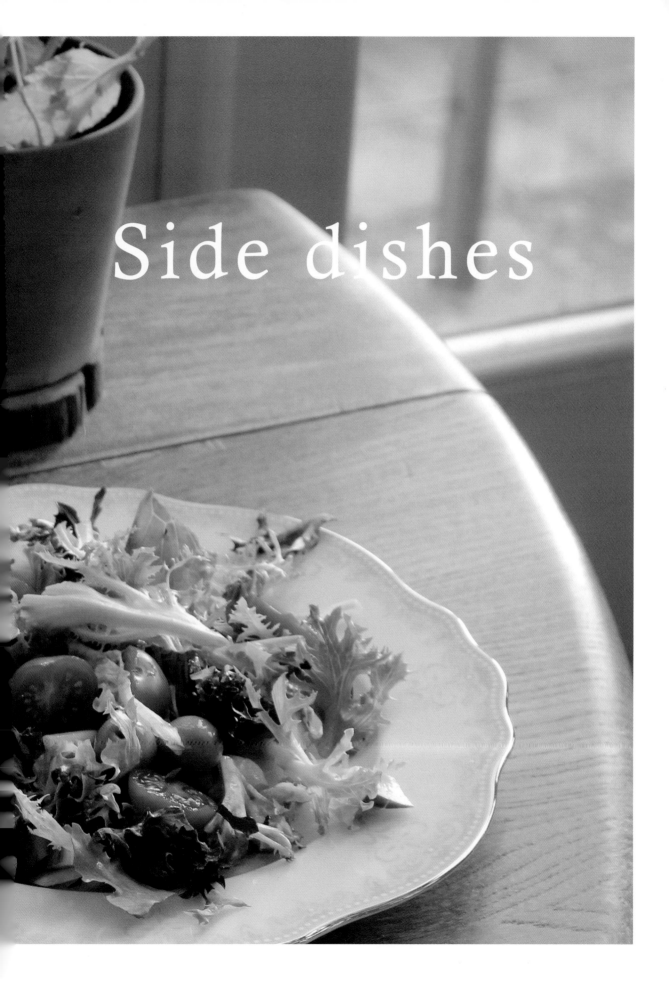

Side dishes

Salads, dressings and sauces

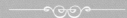

'A big green salad on the side'

You might recognise the expression above from many of the recipes in this book because by having a green salad with every meal you are introducing lots of wonderful enzymes that help break down the other foods. This is a glorious salad which always wins the punters over. Do exclude any ingredients you can't yet have, it will make a wonderful salad either way!

SERVES 2-4

1 heart of Romaine lettuce or 2 heads
of little gem lettuce, chopped
2 cups baby spinach
1 large tomato, chopped or sliced
10 cocktail tomatoes, halved
¼ white cabbage, shredded
2 carrots, grated or chopped
½ cucumber, chopped
½ cup sweet corn
½ red onion, sliced thinly
¼ cantaloupe melon, chopped
or 1 orange, sliced
or 1 apple, chopped
Fresh mint, basil, dill and/
or coriander leaves
A handful of walnuts
Pumpkin seeds and/or sunflower seeds

Mix everything in a bowl and enjoy. Keep any leftovers refrigerated and add to your lunch the next day.

Karen's carrot and pineapple salad

This is a wonderfully refreshing salad, especially lovely for summery garden lunches.

Equal amounts of:
Carrots, grated and
Cabbage, grated and
Fresh pineapple, cubed
Sultanas, a handful – optional
Walnuts, a handful – optional
Juice from ½ lemon

Mix the carrots, cabbage and pineapple and add if you wish the sultanas and/or nuts.

Drizzle lemon juice on top and enjoy.

Cabbage and orange salad

This is a lovely side dish and perfect for a lunch or dinner party.

½ white or red cabbage,
shredded
1 orange, peeled, cut into slices
Chilli flakes, a sprinkling
1 Lime
2 tsp Tamari sauce, or to taste

Shred the cabbage, peel and cut the orange into slices and add to a bowl. Sprinkle chilli flakes on top – more for a spicier version and less for a gentler one. Squeeze the lime juice on top, add the Tamari sauce, mix everything and enjoy!

Veggie medley

1 bok choi head, sliced thinly
1 large carrot, cubed,
sliced or grated
½ cucumber, cubed
1 orange or ½ melon, cubed

Mix all the ingredients and enjoy as they are or with one of the salad dressings on page 154.

Rainbow salad

SERVES: 2

2 heads of little gem lettuce
10 cocktail tomatoes
½ red onion
½ cucumber
1 apple

Shred the gem lettuce, halve the cocktail tomatoes, slice the red onion thinly into half moons, chop the cucumber and cut the apple into chunks. Add everything to a bowl, mix and drizzle with the apple cider vinegar dressing (page 154). Enjoy!

Pretty pomegranate salad

Pomegranate seeds make any salad look and taste wonderful and when married up with tomatoes of all different shapes and colours the results are always absolutely beautiful and delicious. Keep varying the vegetables to create your favourite combinations:

Mixed salad leaves
Cocktail tomatoes – yellow and red, all shapes and sizes
Cucumber, cut into chunks
Red onion, sliced thinly
Carrot, peeled into thin strips
Pomegranate seeds

Place your salad leaves in a beautiful bowl.

Cut up the tomatoes in different ways: slice, chop, halve etc. Place them on top of the salad leaves.

Scatter the red onion and cucumber over the tomatoes.

Pour over the pomegranate seeds.

Serve with your choice of salad dressing, or just as it is.

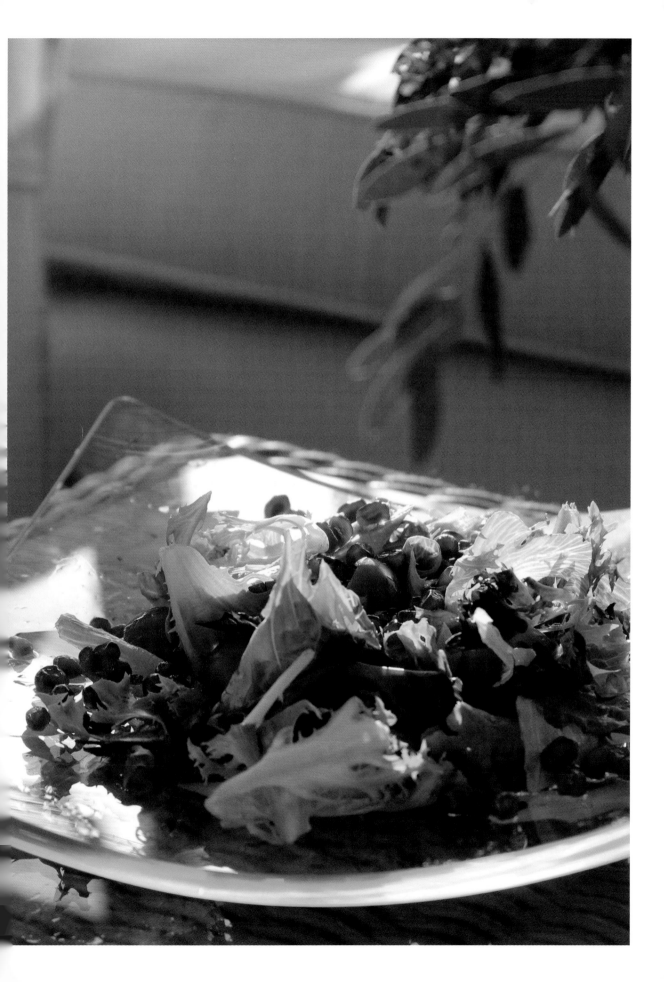

Quinoa, apricot and pine nut salad

This is a delicious dish, where the quinoa takes on the other flavours beautifully.

SERVES: 1

1 cup quinoa
1 cup filtered water
½ tsp lemon juice
Organic herb salt or
Himalayan pink salt
Pine nuts
5 dried apricots, chopped
Black pepper
1 tsp turmeric – optional
Cayenne pepper – optional

Cook the quinoa as per the instructions on the packet, adding the lemon and a dash of organic herb salt or Himalayan pink salt.

Meanwhile, heat a saucepan and add the pine nuts to the dry pan. Keep shaking the pan every now and then until they start getting a touch of colour. Take off the heat, making sure not to burn them.

Stir the apricots and pine nuts into the quinoa and grind some black pepper on top.

Enjoy with, for example, oven-roasted vegetables and a green salad.

If you wish to include the turmeric, just add it to the boiling quinoa.

A sprinkling of cayenne pepper towards the end gives the dish a lovely kick.

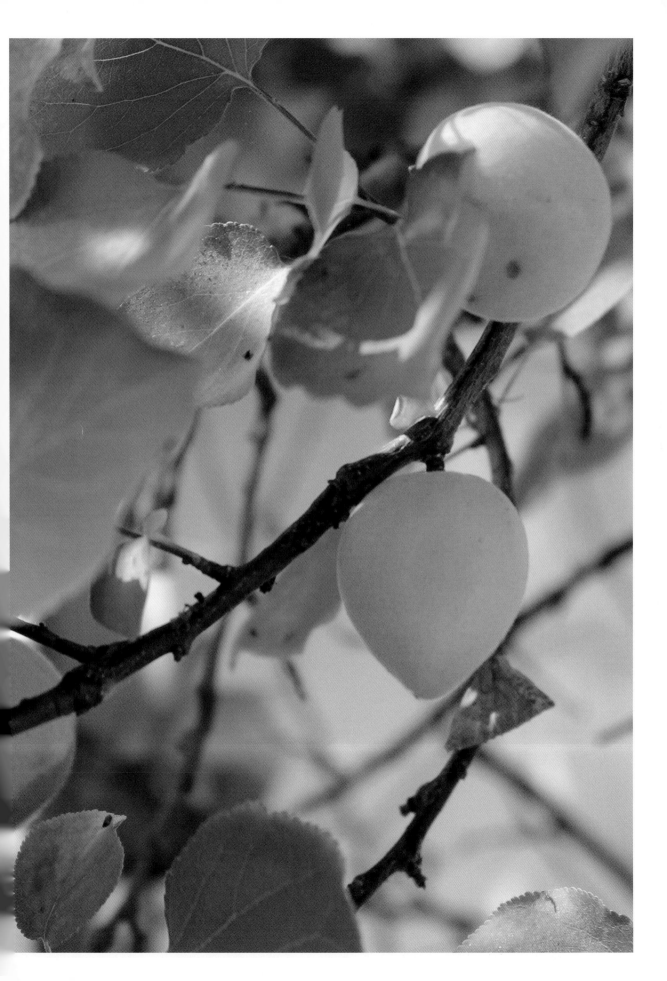

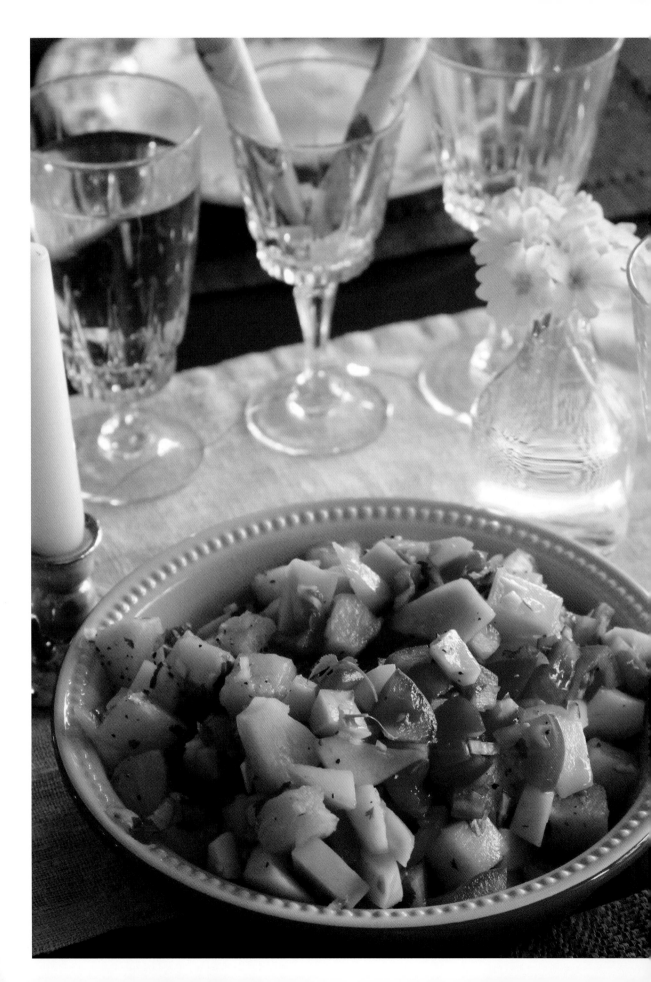

Mango and pineapple salsa

This is a perfect dish on a buffet table
(see the Pretty pomegranate salad on page 145 for another)

SERVES: 6

1 mango, chopped
½ pineapple, chopped
4 large tomatoes and a few
cocktail tomatoes, chopped – do
use tomatoes of all colours and
sizes, the more you mix it up the
more beautiful your salsa will
be!
½ red onion
½ lime
½ red chili, finely chopped –
deseeded or with the seeds in
depending on how hot you like it
Fresh coriander, leaves only
1 tsp maple syrup
Tamari sauce
Black pepper

Mix the mango, pineapple, tomatoes and red onion in a bowl.

Squeeze over the lime, stir in the red chilli, coriander and maple syrup.

Pour on some Tamari sauce and grind black pepper on top.

Taste it until you are happy with how sweet, salty and spicy it is.

Serve with any of the bean or rice dishes, for example.

Garlic-infused spinach

SERVES: 1

1 clove garlic, minced or chopped
2 large handfuls of fresh spinach
¼ tsp Tamari sauce
Black pepper

Warm a pan with a couple of tablespoons of filtered water.

Add the garlic and cook for 30 seconds.

Add the spinach and cook until just wilted – approximately one minute.

Stir in the Tamari sauce and the black pepper.

Transfer to a plate.

Add another dash of water into the hot pan and stir so you get the leftover flavours; then pour over the spinach.

Serve and enjoy.

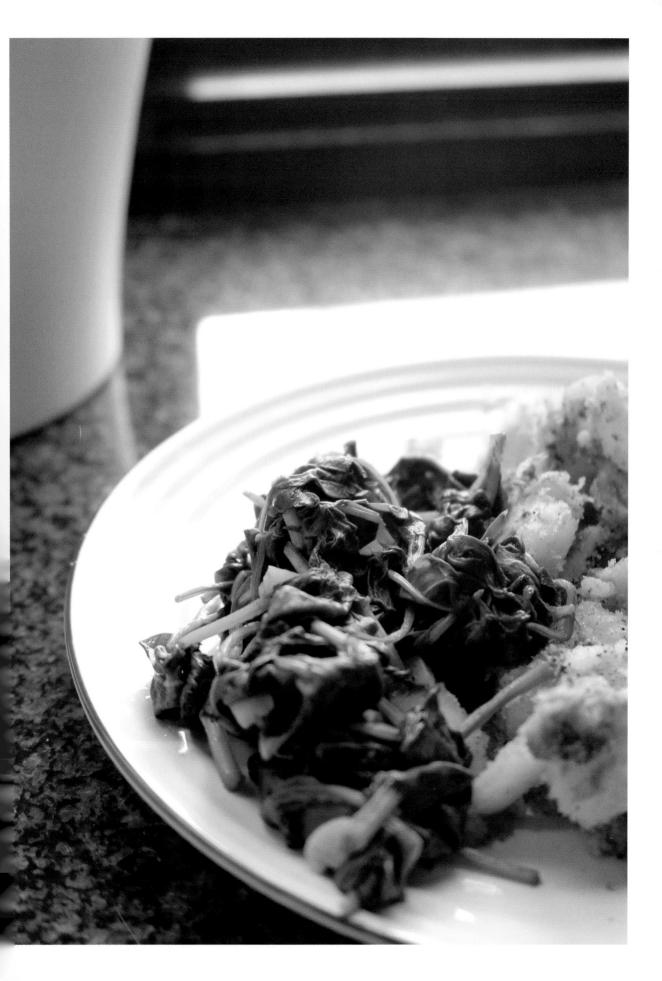

My everyday salad dressing

Some freshly squeezed lemon juice is a simple yet delicious way of dressing a salad.

Apple cider vinegar and orange dressing

This is such a delicious dressing, to which I add maple syrup only on rare occasions.

2 tbsp apple cider vinegar
Juice from ½ orange
(approximately 4 tbsp)
Dried chilli flakes,
a couple of twists
Black pepper, a couple of twists
Organic herb salt, to taste
1 clove garlic, peeled and
crushed with the flat side
of a knife – optional
¼ tsp maple syrup – optional

Stir all the ingredients together and pour over your salad. If you include the garlic, the dressing improves further if you let it infuse for a few hours.

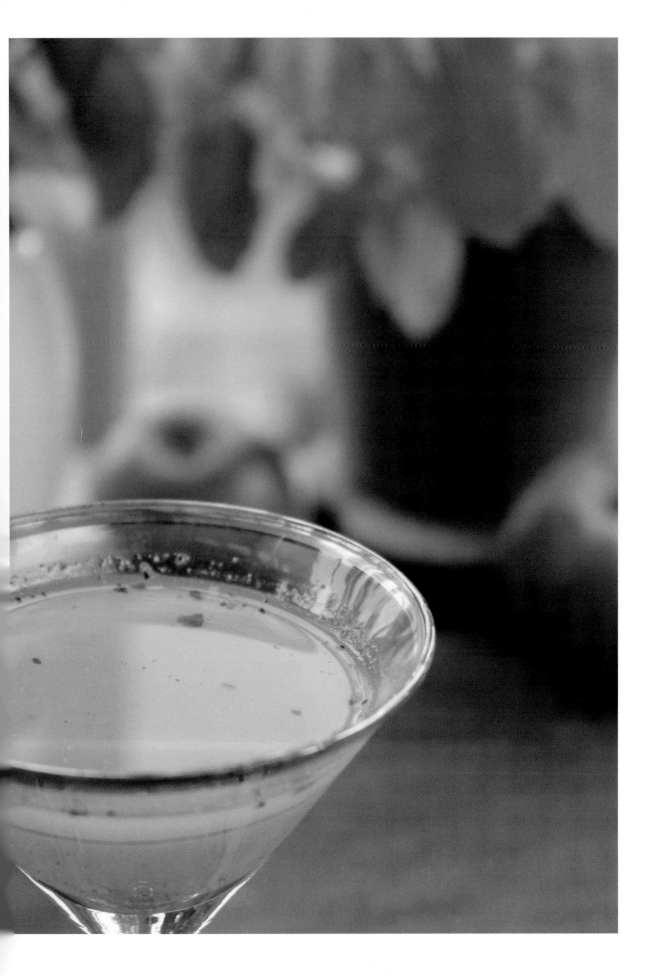

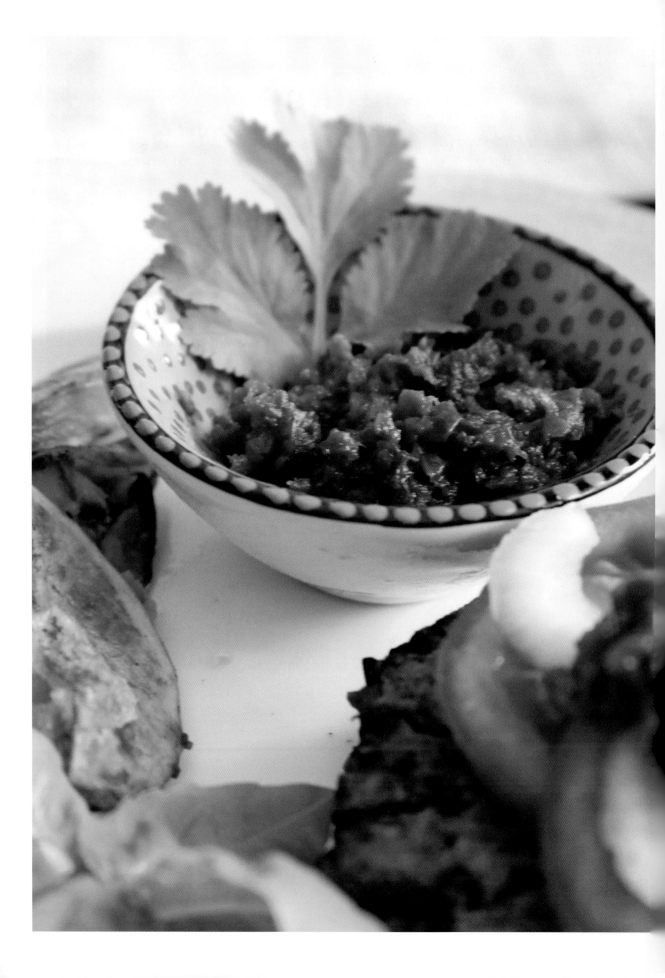

Ketchup

Reserve the water that you soak the sundried tomatoes in (see below), as you will use some of it in this recipe and the rest will go well in tomato sauces and stews.

½ cup dry sundried tomatoes
1½ tsp filtered water from soaking the sundried tomatoes
2 large tomatoes
2 tsp maple syrup
1½ tsp apple cider vinegar
½ tsp Himalayan pink salt
¼ tsp garlic powder

Soak the sundried tomatoes in filtered water for 1-2 hours. You will end up with approximately 1 cup of soaked tomatoes.

Pour off the water into a glass and use in tomato sauces and stews.

Add the fresh and soaked tomatoes to a blender together with the maple syrup, vinegar and seasonings, the small amount of water mentioned in ingredients and blend until smooth.

This is a perfect accompaniment to the Black bean burgers (page 123).

Basil hummus

I use a NutriBullet to blend this hummus; it means pausing on a regular basis to scrape down the sides and stir through with a spoon. A food processor is probably the best option but a regular blender works fine; just add more water if it gets too thick.

1 can of chickpeas or soak ½ cup dried chickpeas overnight and cook as per the instructions on the package
¼ cup lemon juice
1 clove garlic
3 tbsp water, filtered
1 large handful fresh basil leaves
Black pepper
Himalayan pink salt
3 tbsp tahini – optional (remember, this has a high fat content and may be an advanced food for a while)

Blend everything until you are happy with the consistency; add some water if it is too thick.

This is perfect as a snack with some cucumber and carrot sticks or smeared on toast with veggies. I often make hummus for lunch parties as it is perfect for nibbles.

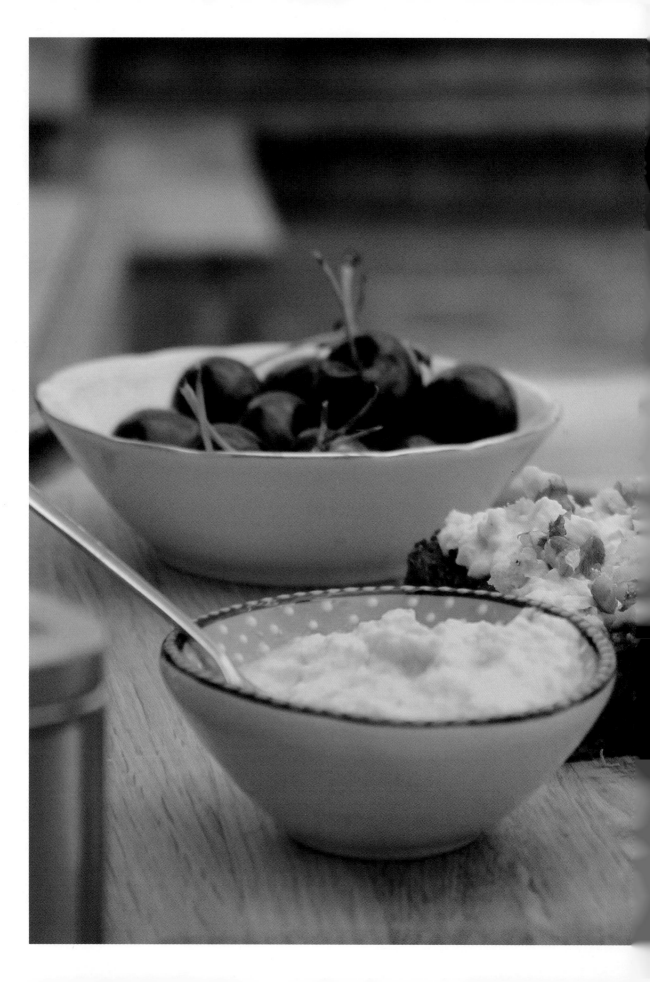

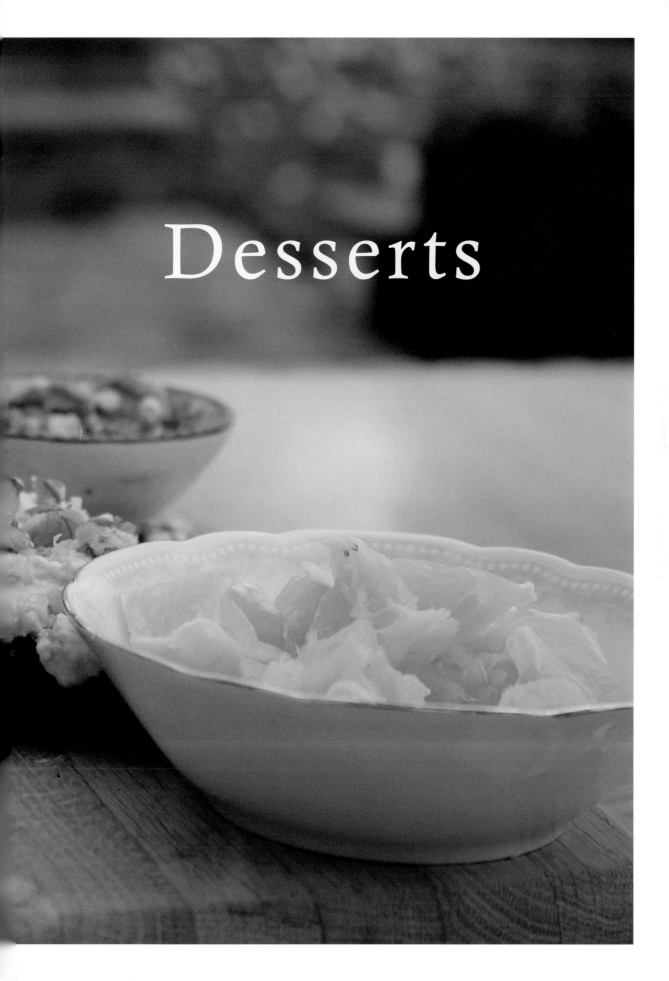

Desserts

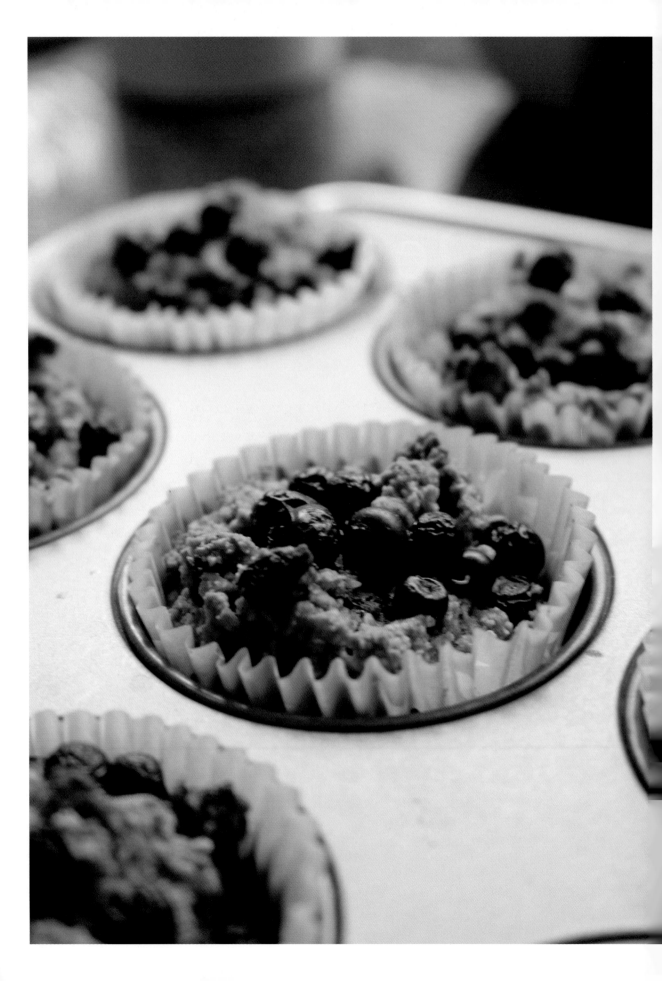

Bakery

Blueberry and raspberry muffins

MAKES 6 MUFFINS

1 cup almond flour
¾ cup oat flour or roughly blended oats
2 tsp baking powder
¾ tsp baking soda
½ tsp Himalayan pink salt
1 tsp vanilla powder
Apple sauce from one apple (see page 50)
2 tbsp maple syrup
¼ cup oat milk
2½ cups fresh raspberries and blueberries mixed

Preheat the oven to 180°C or 350°F (Mark 4).

Mix the dry ingredients.

Mix in the apple sauce, maple syrup and oat milk.

Once you have a smooth batter, fold in the berries carefully and try not to break them.

Spoon the mixture into muffin trays.

Cook in the oven for 25 minutes.

Remove from the oven and leave to cool on a drying rack for approximately 15 minutes.

Enjoy with, for example, a steaming cup of fresh mint tea.

Chocolate brownie

I love desserts that you can eat with a good conscience! To me there is nothing more enjoyable than having a brownie with lots of goodness from the raw cacao and cacao nibs, and natural sweetness from the dates and banana.

4 large dates
2 large ripe bananas
²/₃ cup almond milk
2 tbsp raw cacao
¹/₃ cup gluten-free flour
¹/₃ cup ground almonds
¹/₃ cup desiccated coconut
1 tsp baking soda
¹/₃ cup cacao nibs

The icing:
1 cup dates, pitted
1 tbsp raw cacao powder
¾ cup oat milk (or another plant-based milk of your choice)

The brownie:

Preheat the oven to 180°C or 350°F (Mark 4).

Blend all the ingredients for the brownie except the cacao nibs in a food processor until you have a smooth batter.

Stir in the cacao nibs.

Pour the batter into a non-stick ovenproof dish. A round 23 cm diameter dish is usually a good size but you can make a deeper brownie by using a smaller dish.

Bake in the oven and check how well done it is with a knife after 20 minutes. It should come out slightly gooey and must not get too dry. Once done, take it out and leave to cool down then transfer to a plate.

Serve with coconut yoghurt and fresh berries.

If you wish to make it into a cake, then follow these steps:

The icing:

Add all the ingredients for the icing to a food processor and blend until you have a reasonably smooth texture – if a few chewy bits of dates remain that is perfectly acceptable.

Assembling the cake:

Once the brownie has cooled down, smear the icing on top. You can also decorate with, for example, sliced strawberries, whole raspberries and blueberries.

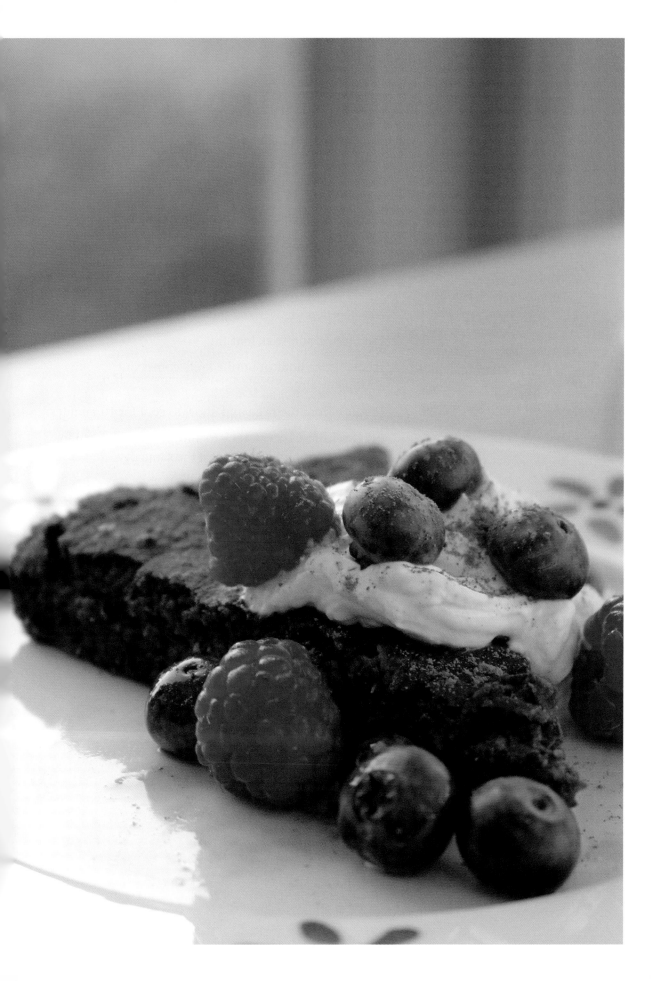

Banana and walnut bread

This bread is heavenly and just as lovely without the walnuts
if you would prefer to leave them out.

1 tsp vanilla powder
2 cups gluten-free flour
¾ tsp baking soda
½ tsp Himalayan pink salt
1 tsp cinnamon, powdered
¼ tsp nutmeg, grated
½ – 1 cup walnuts, chopped
4 bananas, the riper the better
¹/₃ cup oat milk
¼ cup maple syrup
1 tsp apple cider vinegar

Preheat the oven to 180°C or 350°F (Mark 4).

Mix together all the dry ingredients.

In a separate bowl, mash together the bananas, oat milk and maple syrup until you have a smooth consistency.

Mix together the wet and the dry ingredients.

Pour into a non-stick loaf tin.

Bake for one hour or until a knife comes out reasonably clean.

Remove from the oven and allow to cool for 10 minutes.

Flip over onto a metal rack to allow it to cool down for up to an hour and ideally eat it the same day.

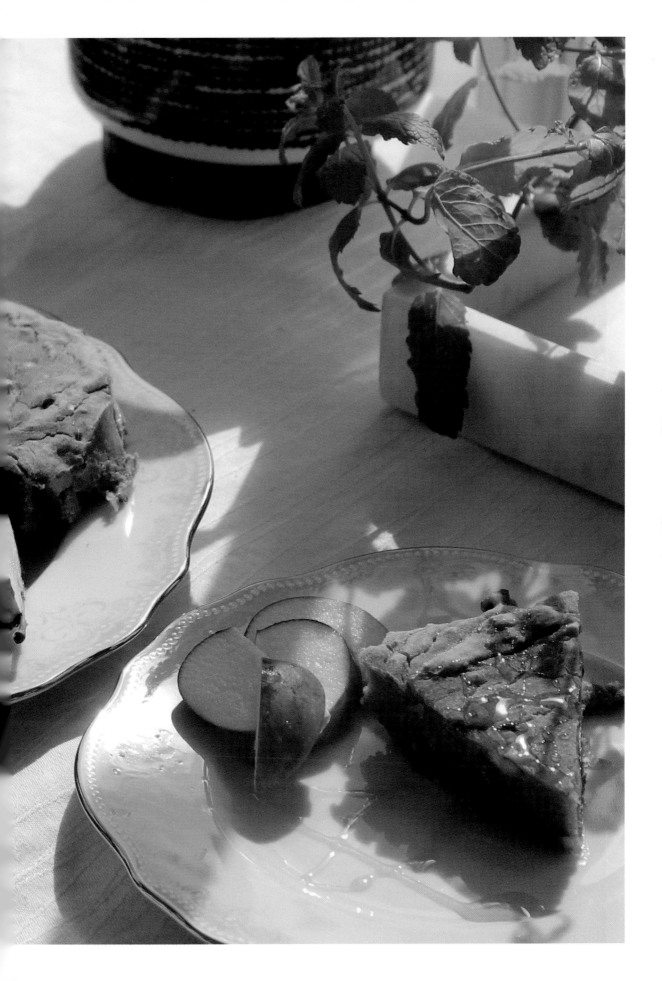

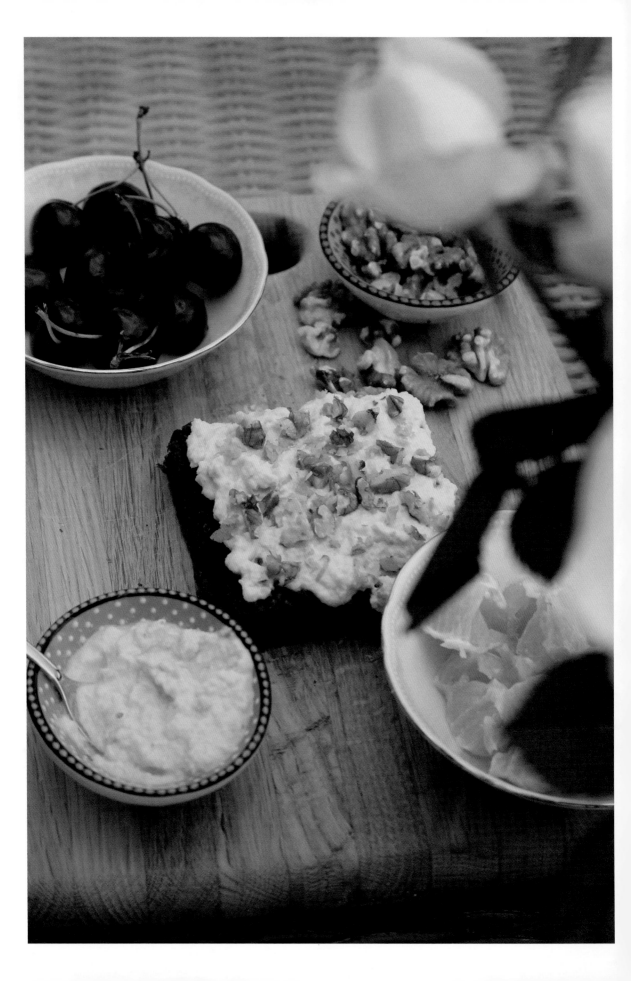

Carrot cake

This is a delicious cake that comes out best when made in a non-stick, oven-proof dish. If you are on the Paddison Program you can exclude the baking powder and baking soda – it is still delicious. Try to soak the cashews overnight beforehand, or for a minimum of two hours. The Nutribullet is a good blender for making the icing. You can make your own oat flour by blending porridge oats for a few seconds.

The cake:

$^1/_3$ cup spelt or gluten-free flour
$^1/_3$ cup almond flour
½ cup oat flour or oats blended
for a few seconds
1 tsp baking powder
1 tsp baking soda
1½ tsp cinnamon, powdered
¼ tsp nutmeg, grated
$^1/_3$ cup maple syrup
1½ cup carrot, finely grated
1 tbsp lemon juice
Apple sauce from one apple
(page 50)

The icing:

1 cup cashews, covered in filtered
water and soaked for at least two
hours
$^1/_3$ cup oat milk
½ tsp vanilla powder
¼ tsp lemon juice
1-2 tsp maple syrup

For decorating the cake:

Grated orange peel from 1
organic, unwaxed orange
A handful of walnuts

Preheat the oven to 180°C or 350°F (Mark 4).

1. The cake

Mix the dry ingredients.

Add the maple syrup, carrots, lemon juice and apple sauce.

Pour into an oven-proof non-stick dish.

Place in the oven for 25 minutes or until a knife comes out clean when you stick it into the centre of the cake.

Remove from the oven and after a few minutes gently turn the oven-proof dish upside down and tip out the cake onto a wire rack and allow to cool.

2. The icing

Drain the cashews.

While the cake is in the oven, add all the icing ingredients to a blender and whiz until you get a smooth consistency.

3. Decorating the cake

When the cake has cooled down, spread the icing on the top and sprinkle the orange peel and walnuts over it.

Serve and enjoy.

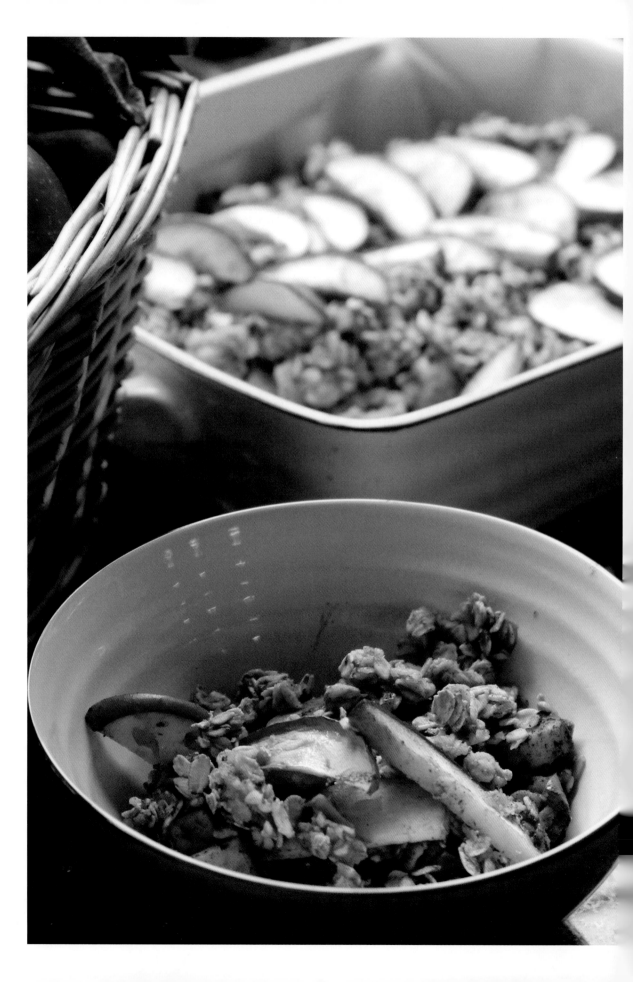

Humble apple crumble

I decided early on to come up with a good crumble recipe as I absolutely love fruit and berry crumbles – the challenge was to think of a way to remove oils and still get a nice texture. The apple sauce gives a helping hand with that and I love how these humble ingredients create such a delicious crumble, which not only makes a great dessert but also doubles up as a comforting and delicious breakfast. I like to leave the skin on the apples for a good intake of fibre and vitamins.

SERVES: 3-4

Crumble:
2 cups rolled oats
½ tsp cinnamon, powdered
A dash Himalayan pink salt
2 tsp maple syrup
½ cup filtered water
½ -1 cup Apple sauce (page 50)
1 handful dried figs or apricots, chopped – optional

Apple filling:
4 cups apples, chopped
2 tsp lemon juice
½ tsp cinnamon
2 tbsp maple syrup + 1 tbsp to drizzle on top

Decoration:
1½ cups apples, sliced

Preheat the oven to 180°C or 350°F (Mark 4).

Combine all the crumble ingredients in a large bowl, including the optional dried figs or apricots, and stir until well mixed.

In a separate bowl, combine all the ingredients for the apple filling except the sliced apples.

Distribute the apple filling evenly on the bottom of an ovenproof dish; I prefer porcelain dishes and have found that no greasing is needed.

Spoon the crumble over the apples.

A lot of cinnamon and maple syrup will be left in the bowl, so add ½ cup of filtered water to the bowl and let it soak up what remains, then pour this mixture evenly over the pie.

Finally, arrange the sliced apples on top, drizzle the last tbsp of maple syrup over it all and bake for 30-40 minutes.

Enjoy as a dessert, snack or breakfast.

Apple crumble with nuts

Once I was able to have nuts I continued to develop the crumble recipe and this is the slightly more advanced version where molasses add a wonderful new depth of flavour.

SERVES: 4-5

Apple filling:
10 large apples
1 tbsp blackstrap molasses
1 tsp cinnamon

Crumble:
1.5 cup nuts, chopped (you can use almonds, pecans, walnuts, cashews etc)
1 cup oats
½ cup gluten-free flour
½ cup desiccated coconut
½ - 1 cup Apple sauce (page 50)

Preheat the oven to 180°C or 350°F (Mark 4).

1. **Apple filling:**

Chop the apples and mix with the molasses and cinnamon in a bowl.

Distribute the apple filling evenly on the bottom of an ovenproof dish, I prefer porcelain dishes and have found that no greasing is needed.

Rinse the bowl with ½ cup water to get all the blackstrap molasses and cinnamon into the dish and pour this over the apples.

2. **Crumble:**

Make the apple sauce and mix with all the ingredients for the crumble in a big bowl. Really work the apple sauce in, as it functions as the oil replacement.

Pour the crumble on top of the apples and rinse the bowl with ½ cup water that you again pour over the crumble.

Place the dish in the oven and cook for 30 minutes.

Serve as is, or with coconut yoghurt. Yum!

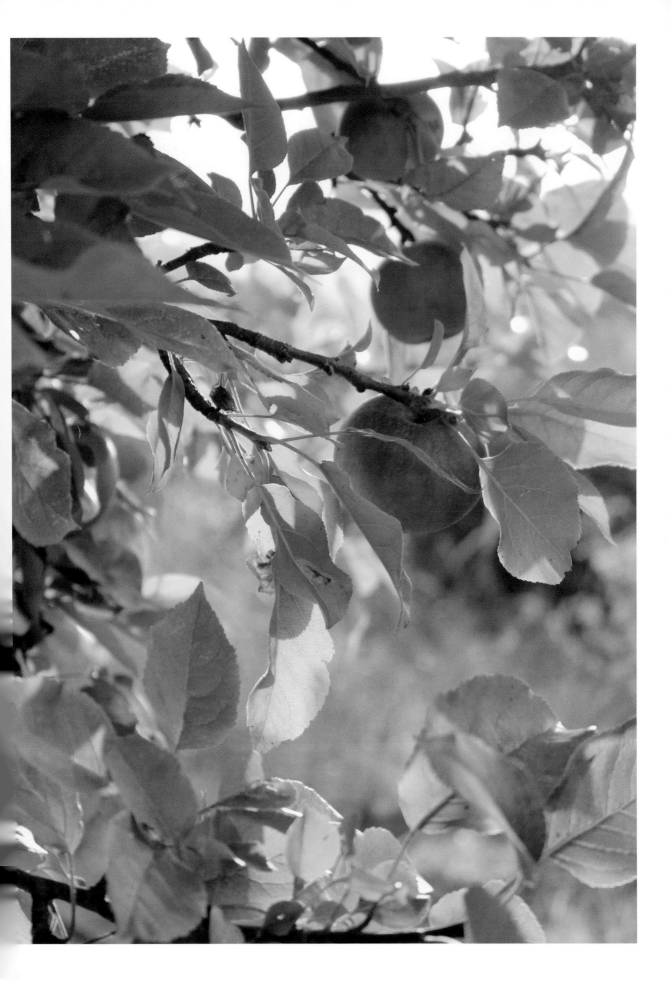

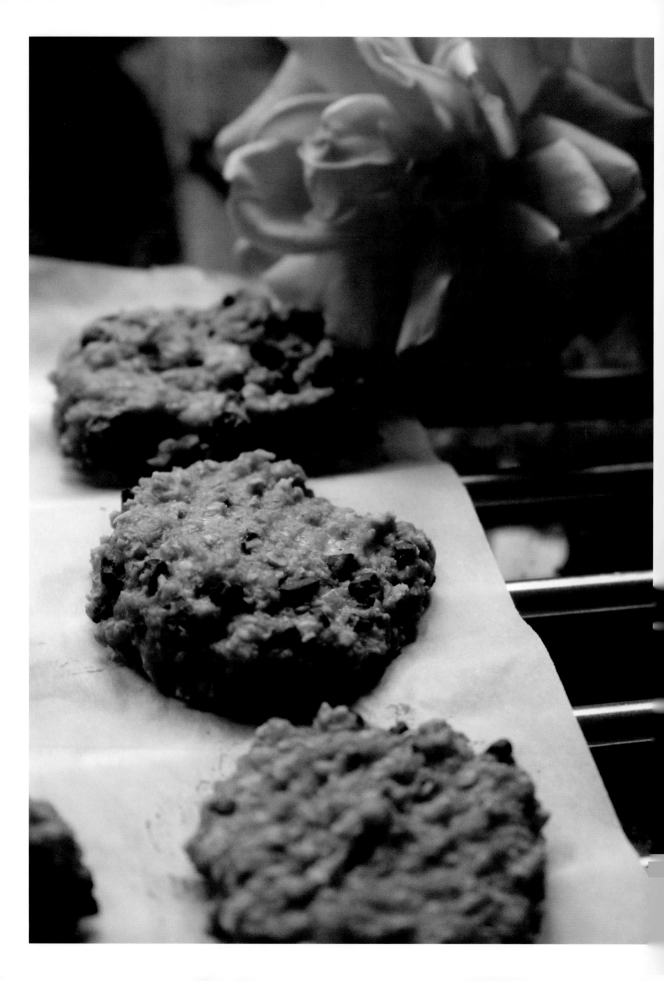

Cacao nib bites

These are so quick and easy to make, with nutritious ingredients, including cacao nibs that you get when the cacao beans are roasted, separated from their husks and broken into smaller pieces. This is the most natural form of chocolate, with very little processing – little power houses of antioxidants, fibre, magnesium and potassium. These 'bites' are perfect as a snack before or after a workout when you want something that gives you energy but doesn't make you feel stuffed and uncomfortable.

⅔ cup gluten-free oats
2 very ripe bananas
1 handful of cacao nibs

Preheat the oven to 180°C or 350°F (Mark 4).

Mix all the ingredients in a bowl, mashing the bananas with a fork.

Make little balls of the 'dough' and place on baking parchment in an oven-proof dish. Either pat them down into flat rounds or keep them as round balls.

Bake in the oven for 20 minutes.

Allow to cool for 15 minutes or until you can't keep your paws off them!

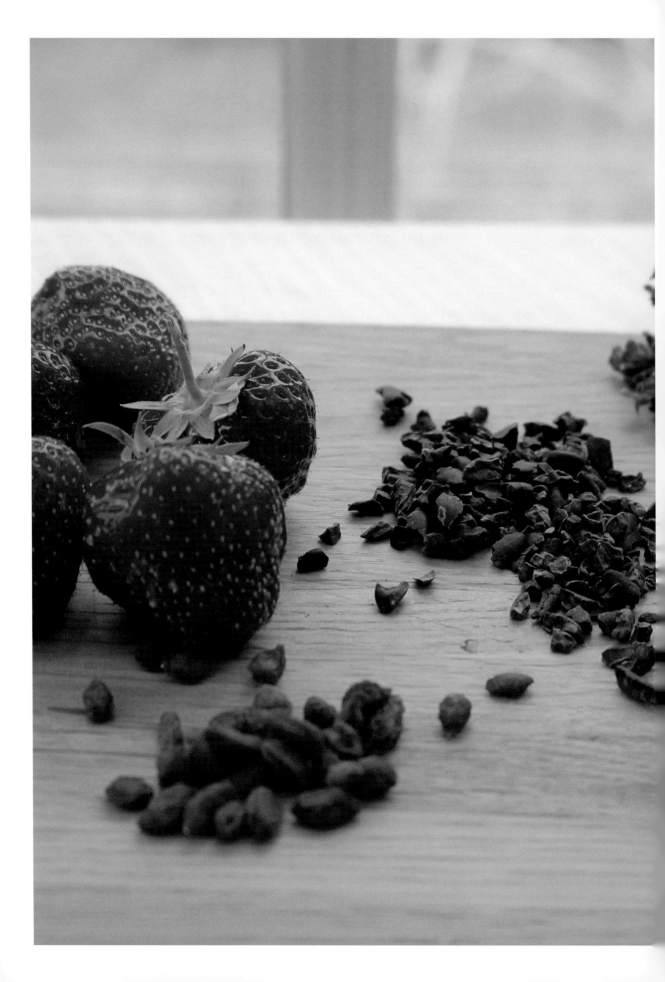

Goji bites

2 very ripe bananas
1/3 cup almond flour
1/3 cup oats
1/3 cut desiccated coconut
1 handful cacao nibs
1 handful goji berries
A dash vanilla powder

Preheat the oven to 180°C or 350°F (Mark 4).

Mix all the ingredients in a bowl. Using a spoon, make six 'cookies' of the dough on baking parchment in an oven-proof dish.

Bake in the oven for 25 minutes.

Allow to cool for 15 minutes and enjoy. They are delicious with some fresh strawberries, which go so well with both bananas and chocolate.

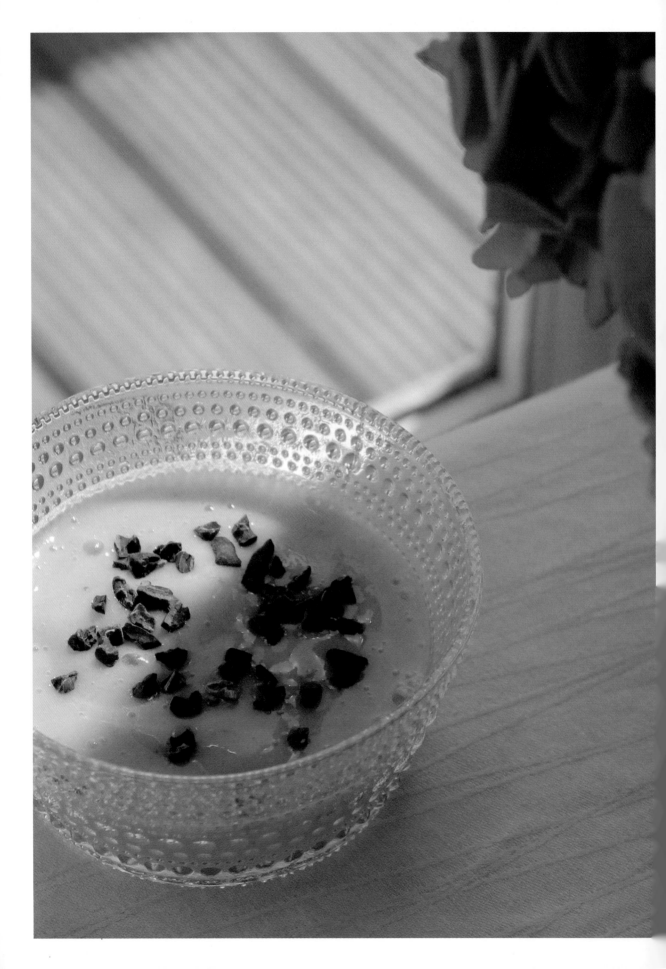

Frozen desserts

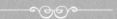

Nice cream

This is a favourite in the plant-based community as it is so delicious, easy to make and full of goodness. You can add all kinds of lovely things here – frozen pieces of fruit, berries, chopped up nuts, cacao nibs... Please note that some blenders may not produce the smoothest results and sometimes you have to add some filtered water, coconut water, oat milk or nut milk to make it perfect, and that is cool too (no pun intended).

SERVES: 1

1 ripe banana
Nut milk or
oat milk – optional

In preparation, take a banana and break it into four pieces. Place the pieces in a freezer bag or Tupperware container in the freezer for at least two hours.

Once the banana is frozen, place the pieces in your blender and whiz until you have a smooth consistency.

Serve and enjoy.

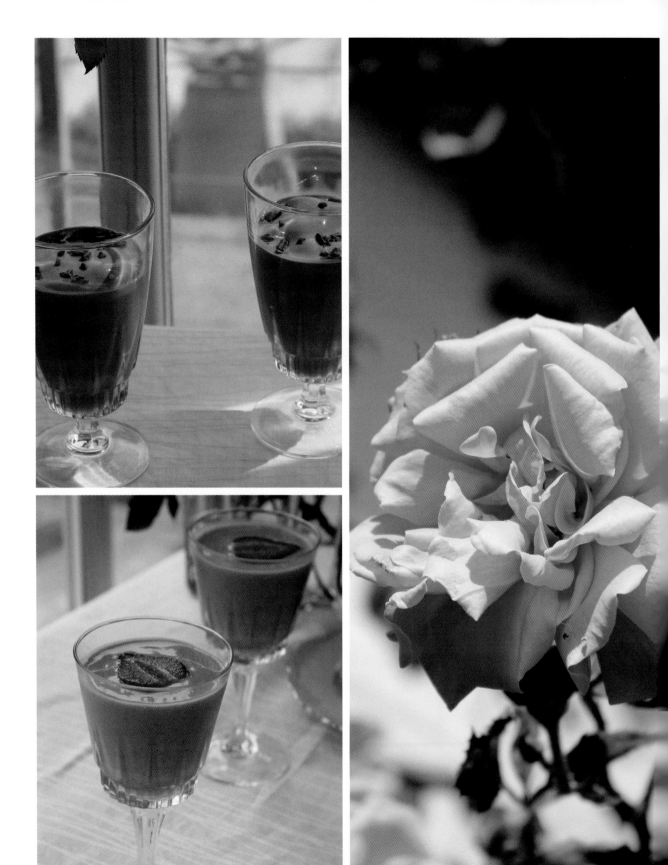

Chocolate shake

This is the most delicious, creamy, chocolatey shake that you could ever wish for and the little cacao nibs add a delightful crunch. A great tip is always to keep peeled, chopped bananas in the freezer – frozen banana goes so beautifully in smoothies, shakes and nice cream.

SERVES: 2

2 frozen bananas, peeled and frozen in pieces
¾ cup cashew, almond or oat milk
2 tbsp raw cacao powder
Handful cacao nibs
Dried goji berries – optional

Blend the bananas, plant-based milk and cacao powder until smooth. If it becomes too thick to blend, just scrape the sides of the blender cup/bowl with a spoon, stir through and keep blending until you have your perfect consistency. Add more liquid if necessary.

Pour into glasses and sprinkle the cacao nibs on the top.

Goji berries are also delicious sprinkled on the top.

Enjoy through a thick straw.

Strawberry shake

SERVES: 2

2 frozen bananas, peeled and frozen in pieces
¾ cup cashew or almond milk
2 cups strawberries
Handful cacao nibs or 1 sliced strawberry – optional for decoration

Blend the bananas, nut milk and strawberries until smooth.

Pour into glasses and sprinkle the cacao nibs or sliced strawberries on top.

Serve through a thick straw.

Fruit and berries

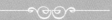

Frozen watermelon

Let's not underestimate the beauty of a simple dessert like frozen watermelon. We had it while travelling around the Southern Cape and it was the most delicious and refreshing treat in the sweltering South African sun.

1 watermelon

Cut the watermelon into 2 cm-wide pieces, leaving the skin on.

Put the pieces in a freezer-proof container, place in the freezer for 1-2 hours, until lightly frozen.

Let everybody grab their own piece(s) and enjoy.

Passion fruit-glazed fruit salad

Select your favourite fruit, for example:

Papaya
Mango
Pineapple
Oranges
Apples
Banana
Grapes

Passion fruit is essential

Chop everything and mix all except the passion fruit in a large bowl.

Spoon in the passion fruit and stir through.

Serve and enjoy.

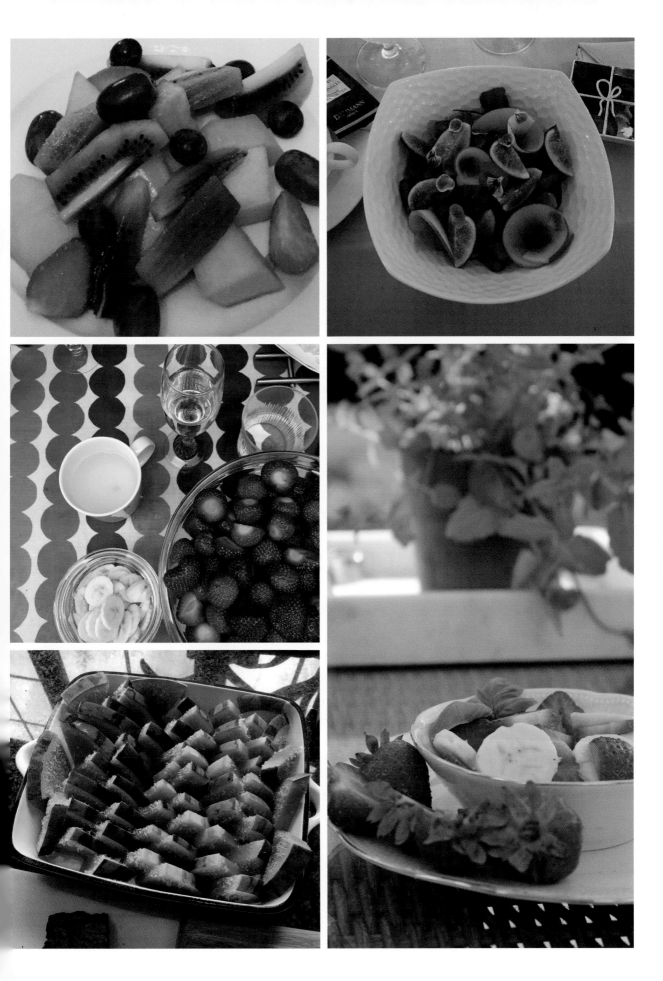

Strawberries and oranges

Strawberries, sliced
Oranges, peeled and cut into smaller pieces

Strawberries and oranges go so well together, this is one of my favourite summery desserts.

Strawberries and bananas

Strawberries, sliced
Bananas, sliced

Place in a bowl and enjoy – these flavours are a match made in heaven.

For the love of raspberries and lime

SERVES: 2

2 cups raspberries, washed

Sauce:
1 lime, halved
1 tsp maple syrup
Mint leaves

Place the raspberries in a bowl.

In a separate bowl, stir together the lime and maple syrup. Keep adding maple syrup until you are happy with the sweetness.

Stir the sauce into the raspberries and serve with a mint leaf on top.

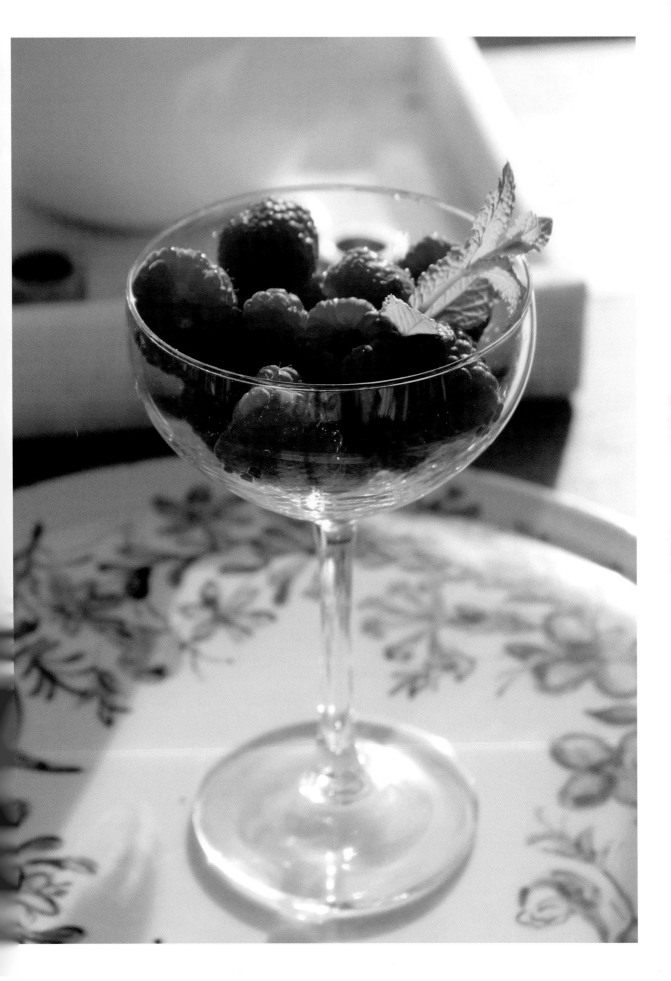

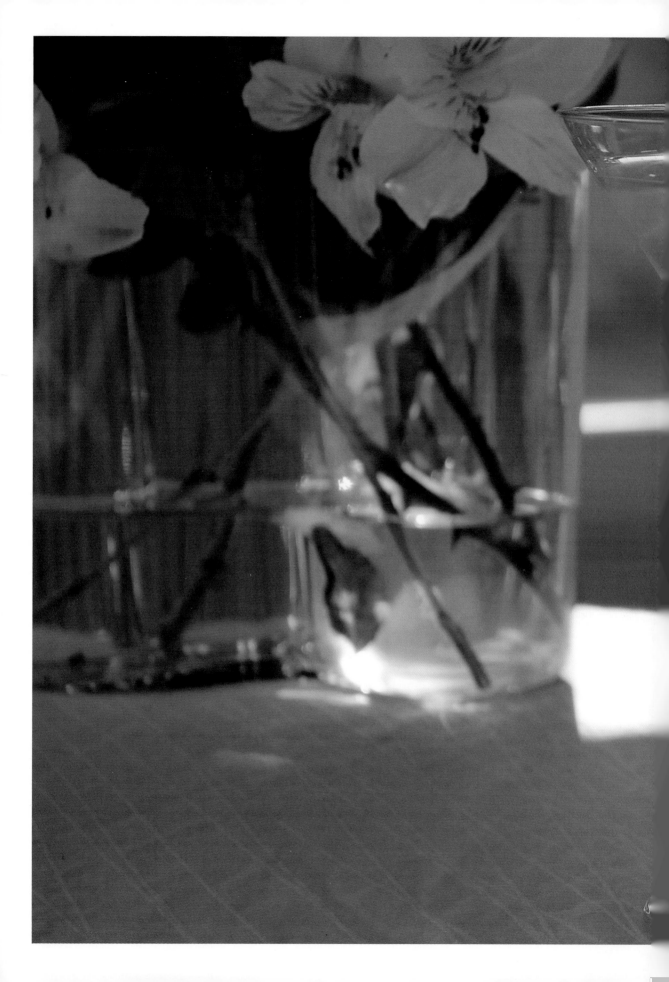

Drinks

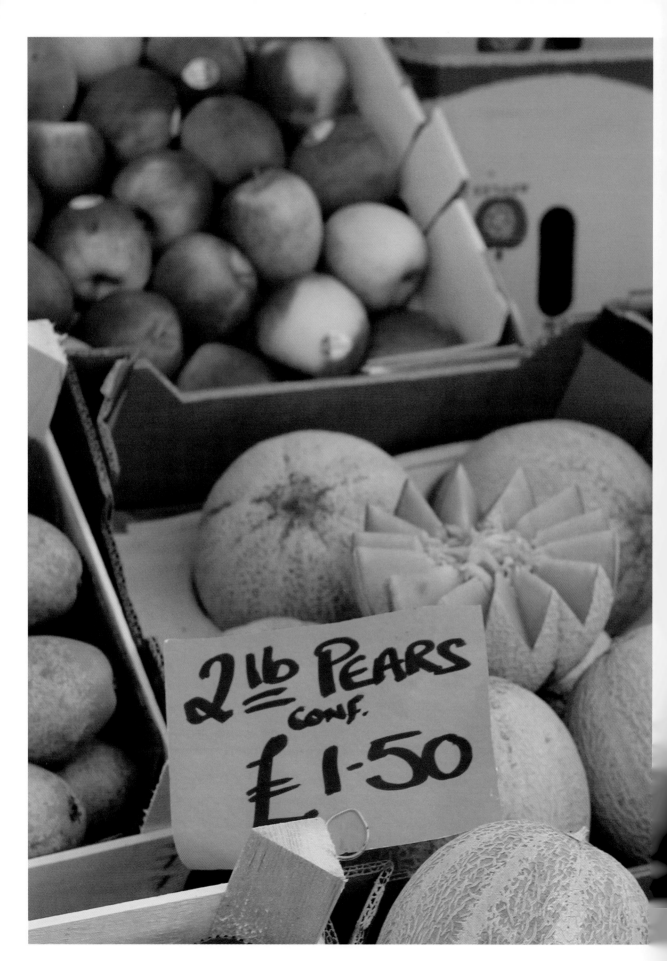

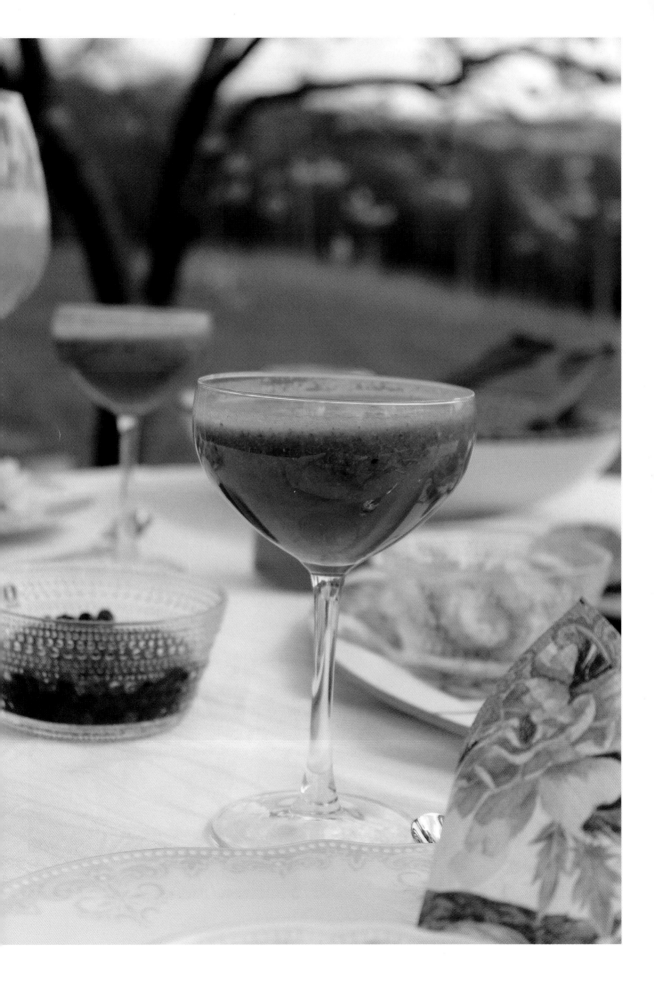

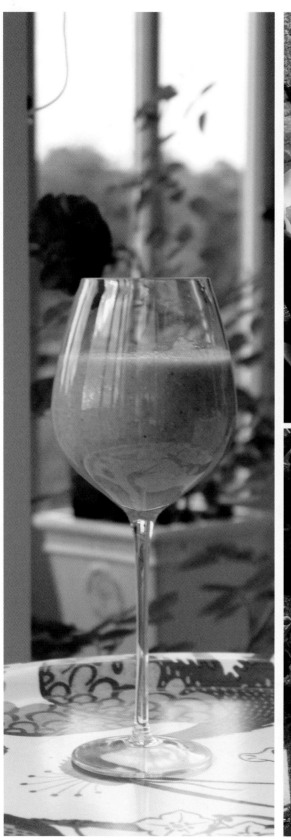
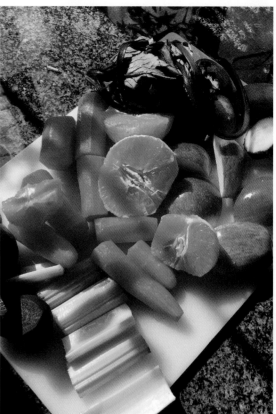
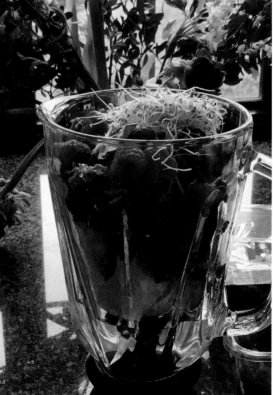

Smoothies

I love my smoothies and when friends and family come to stay with me they always get to wake up to a green, red, black or orange smoothie.

There is nothing better than flooding your system with happy vitamins and minerals first thing in the morning, as they set you up for the day ahead. In fact, my diligent smoothie drinking might very well be one of the reasons why I didn't develop a worse version of rheumatoid arthritis (page 13), so I would really encourage you to implement this delightful detail into your daily routine.

Here are a few recipes to start you off, before you go free-styling and making up your own favourites. Always make sure to include as much green vegetable as possible, because fruit is yummy but also comes with a lot of sugar, so you want to go stronger on the veggies. It might take you a few weeks to get used to having smoothies so don't be too hard on yourself but allow some extra fruit in there in the beginning; then gradually reduce the amount. If your smoothie is too bitter, just add some banana, as it always takes the edge off very intense veggie flavours.

I prefer to have my smoothies as soon as possible after making them, as they don't taste as nice after a few hours. Another tip is always to have some frozen chopped banana available, as it gives smoothies such a creamy texture, chills them perfectly and makes them taste just delicious.

Everyday beauty greens

SERVES: 1

1 large handful of spinach or kale
1 orange
½ cup filtered water

Keep it simple folks – just blend all of this and you have a wonderful start to your day.

To this smoothie you can just add any fruits or vegetables; the following are some of my favourites:

Fresh ginger
Cucumber
Courgette
Banana

Prettifying pineapple

SERVES: 1

1 thick slice of fresh pineapple
½ banana
1 handful of spinach or kale
½ cup filtered water

Blend all the ingredients together and enjoy.

The micronutrient bromelain in the pineapple is anti-inflammatory and also helps with digestion.

The frozen smoothie

A bag of lettuce that is just too sad to serve as salad can make the perfect smoothie ingredient. The frozen banana and pineapple give the smoothie a creamy texture in addition to a lovely flavour.

SERVES: 1

1 thick slice of courgette
A handful of spinach
A handful of mixed lettuce
½ frozen banana
½ cup frozen pineapple
½ orange

Blend all the ingredients together and enjoy.

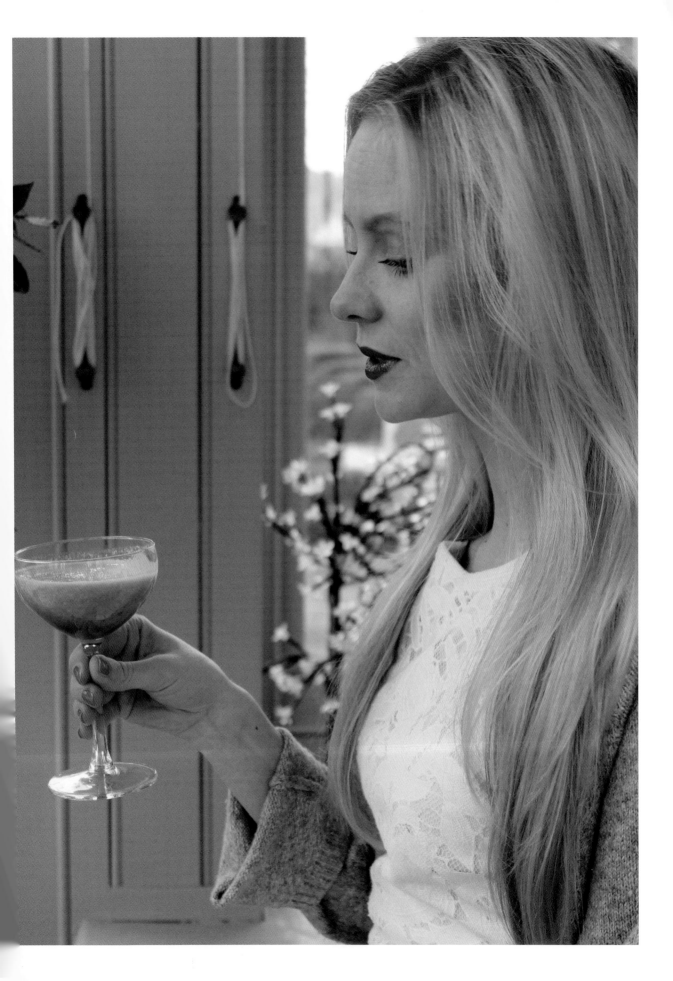

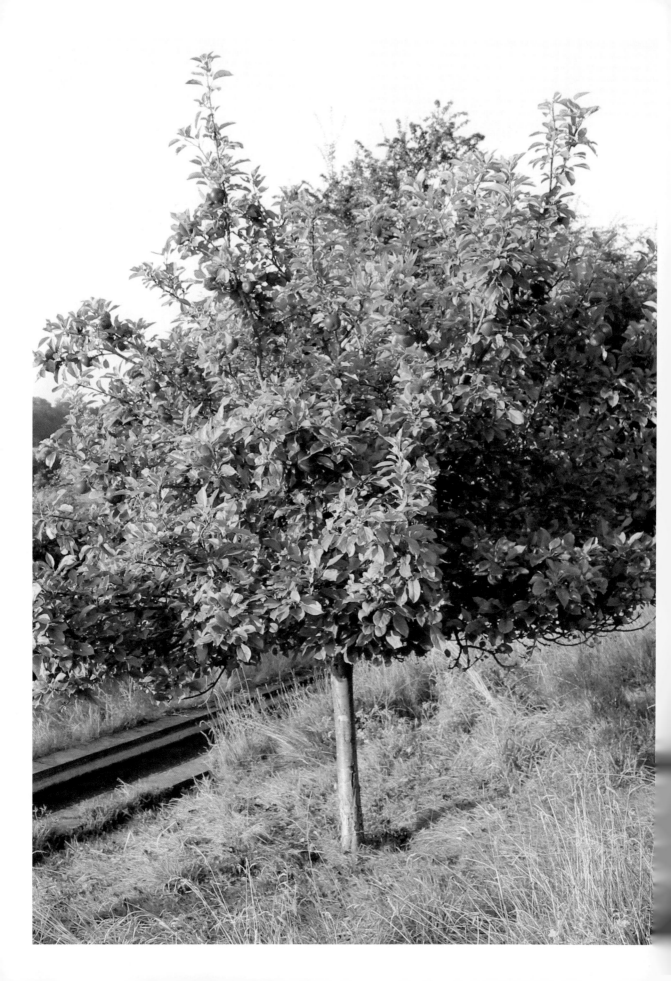

The whole garden smoothie

This smoothie illustrates that you can take whatever you have in your kitchen or growing in your garden and combine it to make a most delicious smoothie.

SERVES: 2-3 PEOPLE

1 handful of kale
4 large leaves of Swiss chard
2 cm fresh ginger
1 beetroot (red or yellow)
1 pear
1 kiwi
1 banana
½ cup oat milk or filtered water

Blend everything together and enjoy.

The midnight smoothie

The blackberries give this smoothie the most splendid vibrant dark colour.

SERVES: 1

1 handful of spinach
5 blackberries
½ banana
1 orange
½ cup filtered water

Blend all the ingredients together and enjoy.

The who-needs-a-milkshake-anyway smoothie

This is more of a dessert smoothie with its creamy texture and delicious flavour.

1 cup almond milk
3 large strawberries
½ banana
1 handful of spinach
1 tsp cinnamon

Blend all the ingredients together and enjoy.

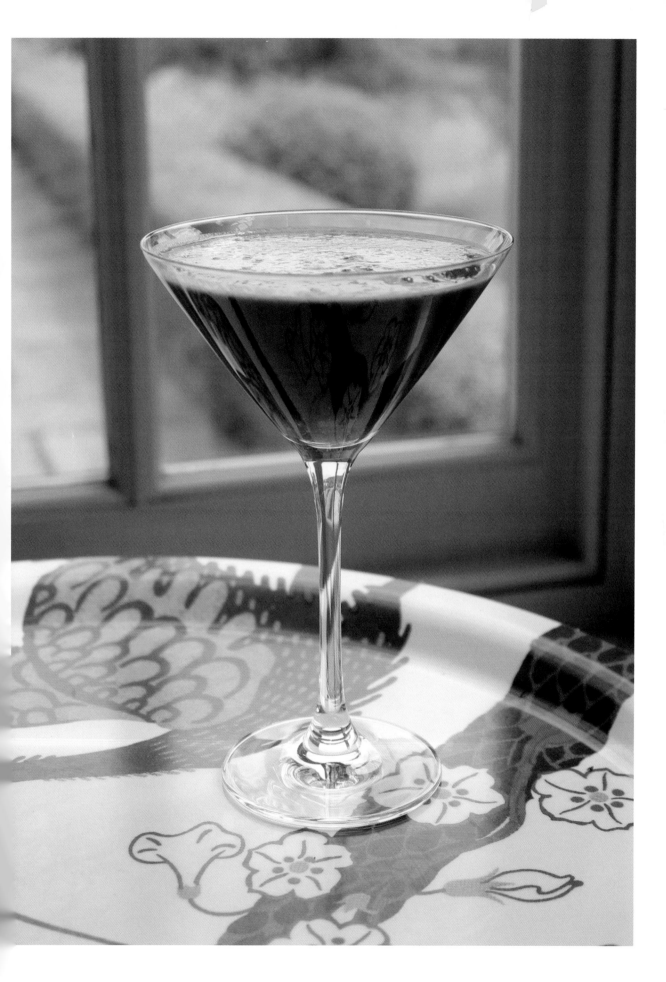

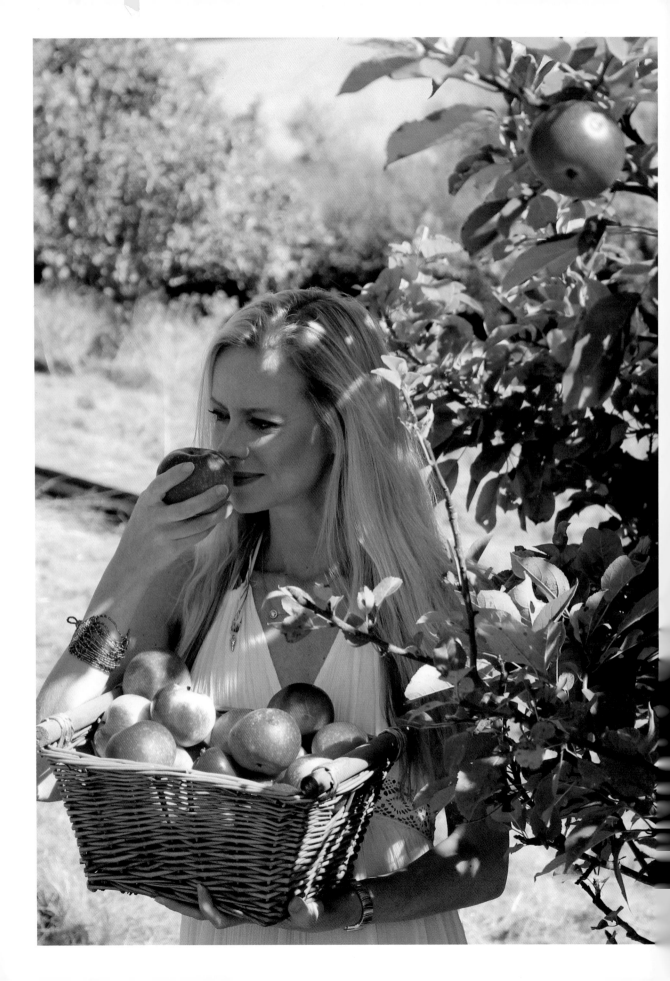

Juices

I bought a juicer when I started the Paddison Program (page 14) and these days I just love juicing all kinds of vegetables and fruits and it is such fun to mix and match wildly to see what delicious flavour combinations there are.

Apple juice

When I moved to the country I discovered that there were lots of apple trees in my garden, so I have had to learn to make compotes and juices on a grand scale. Fortunately, apple juice is delicious, and very easy to make:

SERVES: 1

2 large apples

Cut the apples into four chunks. Discard the core but keep the skin on, place in the juicer and juice into the most delicious apple juice.

Fresh orange juice

Nothing beats freshly pressed orange juice. Just peel three oranges, put them in your juicer and whizz it up.

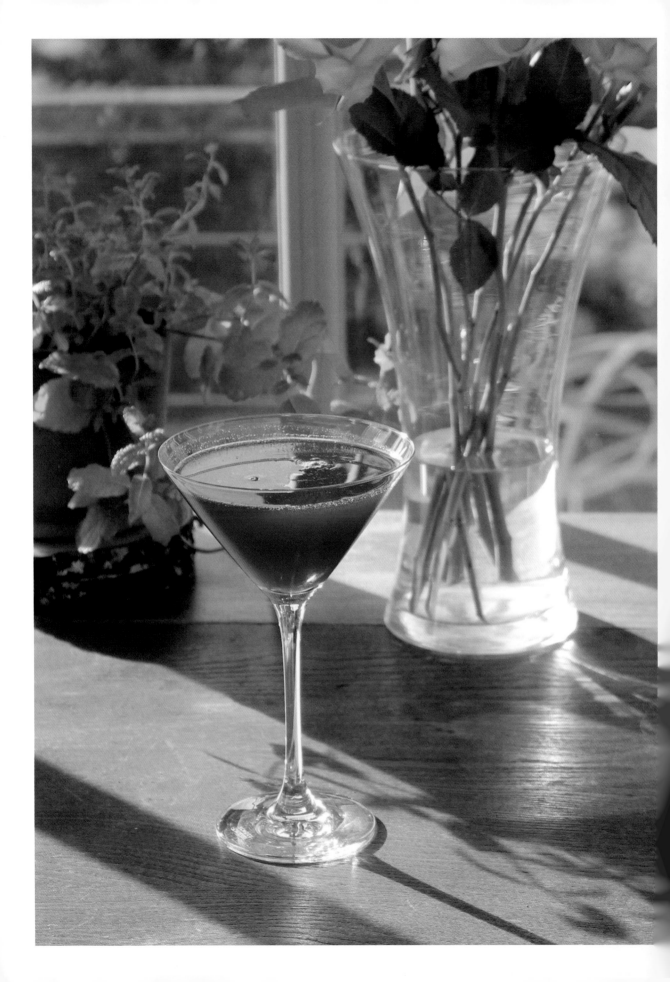

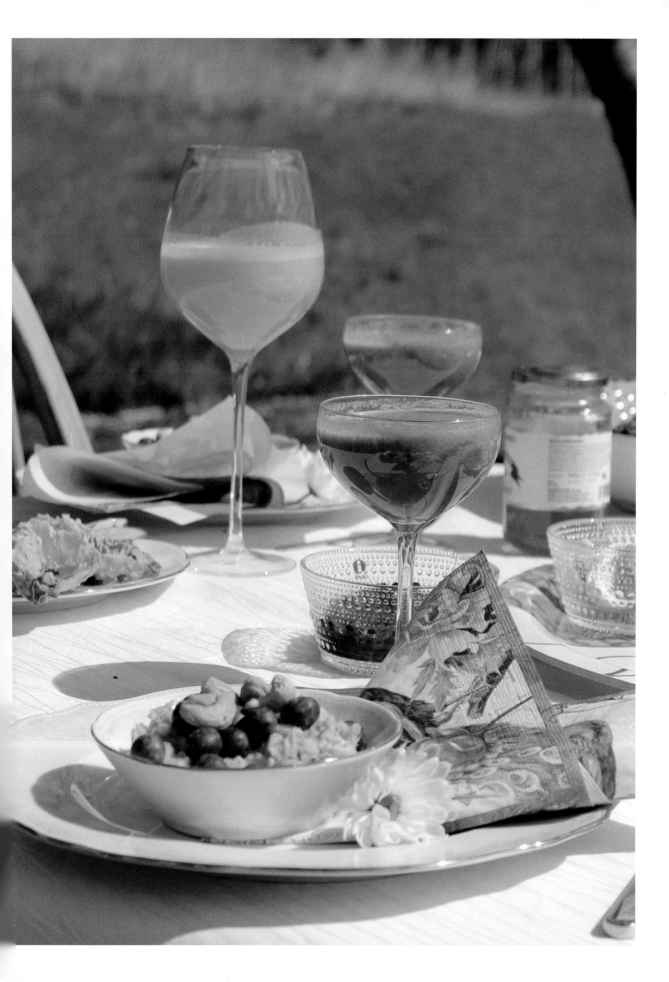

Garden delight juice

1 carrot
1 celery stalk
1 beetroot
1 apple
2 oranges
10 cm chunk of cucumber

Juice it all up and enjoy.

Watermelon juice

Sometimes when buying a watermelon I have found that there is just SO much of it that it is impossible to get through it all. Well, juicing it is the best way to avoid wasting it, so just pop the pieces in your juicer and enjoy. Watermelon juice is especially perfect for parties – just remember to leave a few pieces of the fruit to decorate the drinks.

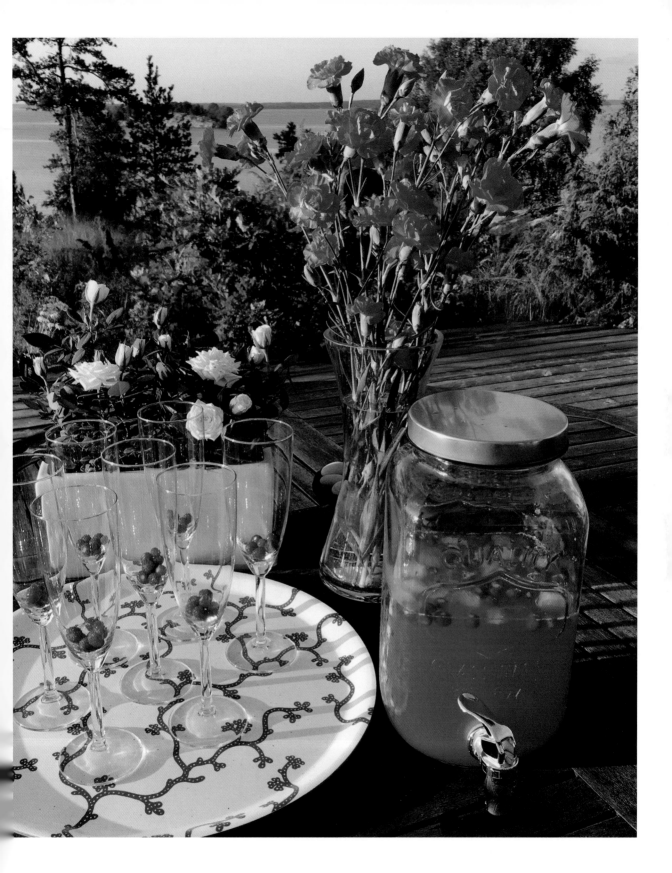

Cold drinks

I haven't had any alcohol since I started on the Paddison Program and I can tell you that it is the one thing that I miss the least. However, at social occasions it is nice to have a drink in your hand, so I tend to go for one of the following:

Coconut water

Coconut water is a delicious drink which also contains a wealth of vitamins and helps fight free radicals that are known to cause damage in our bodies. If you do not have fresh coconuts from which to extract it, the unpasteurised, raw packaged versions are the ones to go for, as they contain all the possible nutrients. There are lots of pasteurised versions available but in the process the coconut water is heated to 63° C (145° F) for 30 minutes to kill off bacteria and to extend shelf life, which strips it of some of its vitamins. If you cannot find raw coconut water, do keep an eye out for some that has undergone High Pressure Processing (HPP), where the bacteria are killed off and the shelf life is prolonged, but where the nutrients are kept intact.

Lemon water

This is considered to be a 'beauty drink' where you squeeze the lemon into some lukewarm water for the best start to your day. Have it 15 minutes before breakfast, as it kick-starts your digestion, helps fight infection and has strong antibacterial and antiviral powers.

Sparkling water... with slices of:

Lemon or
Lime or
Lemon and cucumber or

Strawberries or
Pomegranate seeds

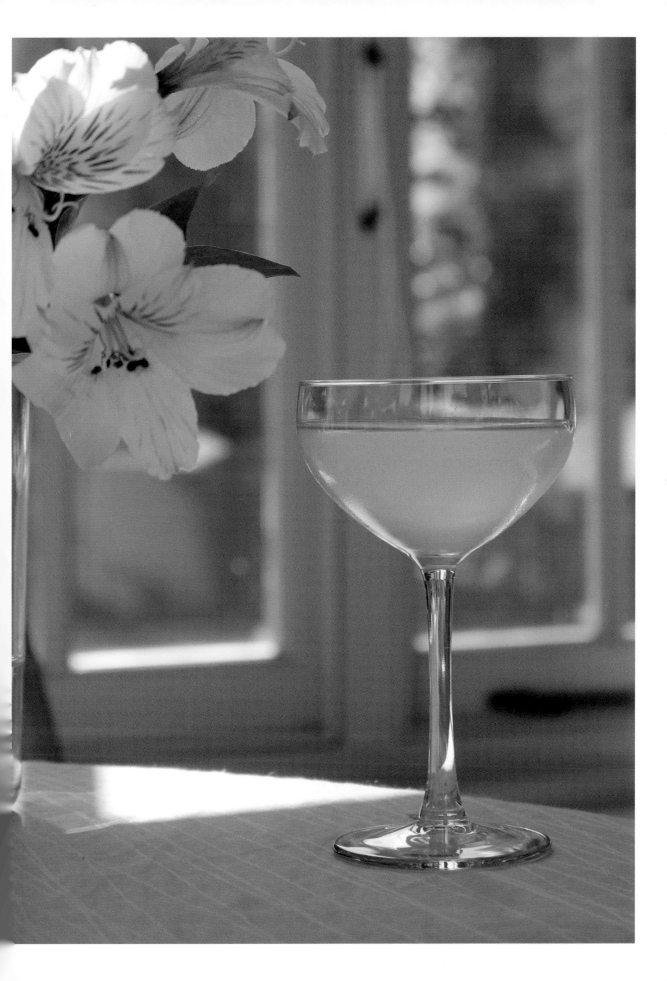

Hot drinks

I no longer drink black tea or coffee, but the winters here in England can get very cold and rugged so I do still enjoy a hot drink every now and then and these have become my favourites:

Fresh mint tea

These days I always keep a bunch of fresh mint (spearmint/peppermint/apple mint – try different ones and find your favourites) in a mug of water in the fridge. It is so easy just to boil some water, place the mint in a mug, pour over the water and enjoy the most delightful cup of fresh mint tea.

Hot lemon and ginger

This is another lovely hot drink that is perfect during the winter months or if you have a cold. Just mix the juice from half a lemon with a few slices of fresh ginger in a mug of hot water, allow to infuse for four minutes, then enjoy. You can always add ½ tsp of maple syrup if you wish to make it sweeter.

Rooibos

This is a wonderful South African red bush herb, which contains loads of minerals and antioxidants and is known to be anti-inflammatory.

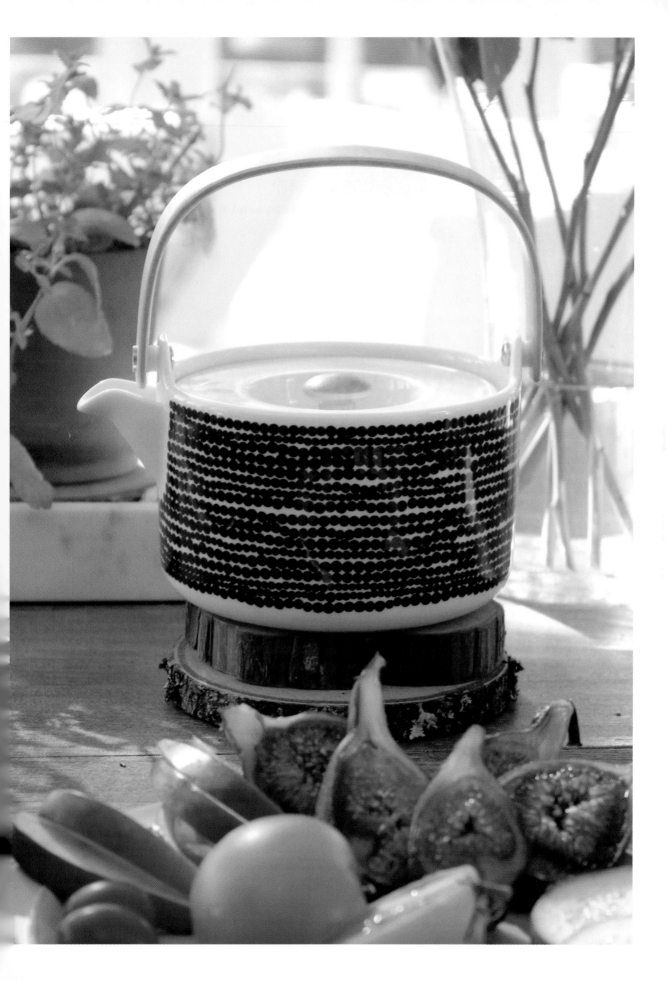

Hot chocolate

SERVES: 1

*1 tbsp unsweetened
raw cacao powder
1-2 dates, depending on how
sweet you like it
1 cup oat milk*

Add all the ingredients to your blender and whizz until you have a smooth drink.

Pour into a saucepan and warm up but do not bring to the boil.

Serve and enjoy.

Pumpkin potion

This is a perfect drink to make when you have leftover steamed pumpkin from other dishes. It is such a warming hot drink, perfect during the colder months and the scent of cinnamon that fills the house is just divine.

SERVES: 1

*1 cup oat milk
2 tbsp steamed pumpkin
¼ - ½ tsp cinnamon
⅛ tsp nutmeg
½ tsp vanilla powder
1 tsp maple syrup
A dash of cayenne pepper*

Add all the ingredients to your blender and blitz until you have a smooth drink.

Pour into a small saucepan and heat gently, stirring occasionally. When it is just about to start boiling, remove from the heat and serve in your favourite mug.

Best enjoyed all snuggled up under a blanket with a good book.

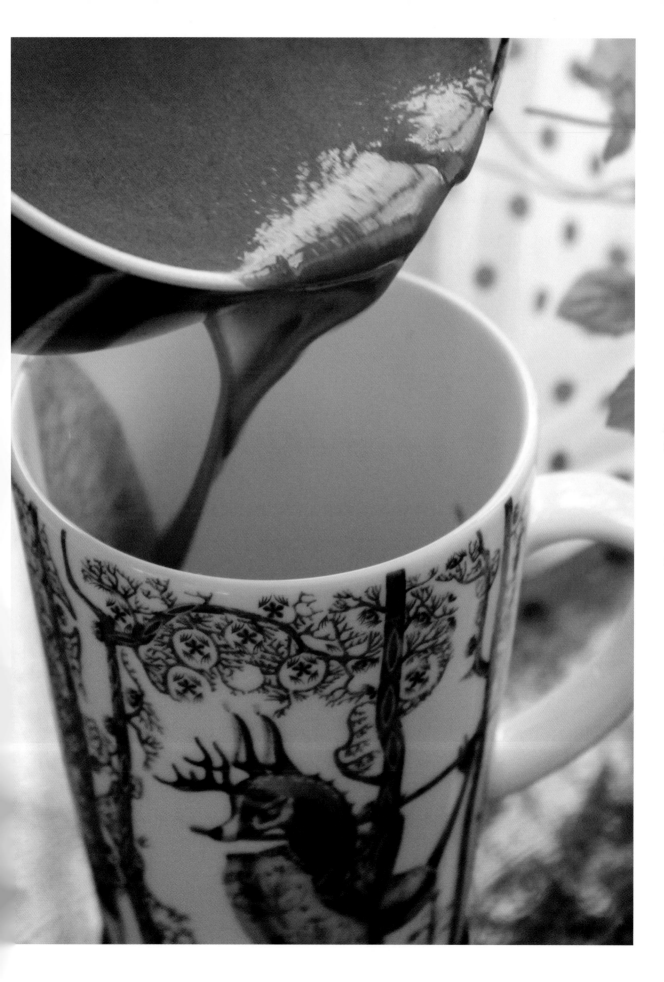

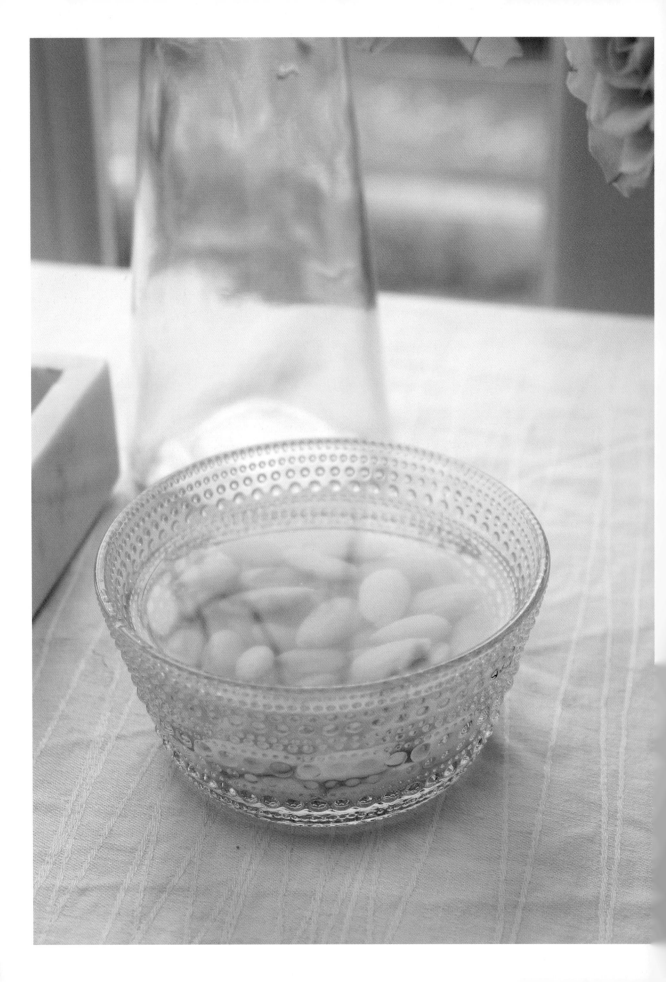

Plant-based milk

⟡

Plant-based milk is very rewarding to make at home and especially delicious in smoothies or porridge, where it creates a really creamy consistency. Soaking the nuts in water overnight will make them easier to digest, so don't skip this step.

Almond milk

1 cup raw organic almonds
3 cups of filtered water

Soak the almonds in a bowl of filtered water overnight, or for a minimum of four hours. Drain.

Place the almonds in a blender with the water and blend for about a minute until the consistency is milky.

Strain the almond milk through a nut milk bag or a muslin bag into a glass bottle using a funnel.

Almond milk keeps in the fridge for three to four days.

I sometimes peel the almonds before blending, which is somewhat time consuming but means you can skip straining the almonds and thereby be sure to retain all the vitamins and minerals found in the nuts. The consistency will be grainy but when used, for example, to make creamy porridge you won't even notice it.

To peel the almonds you will first need to submerge them in boiling water for 10 seconds, then plunge them into cold water. They can then be peeled easily as they will come shooting out of their skins when given a little twist.

A sprinkling of cinnamon or vanilla adds a lovely variation of flavour.

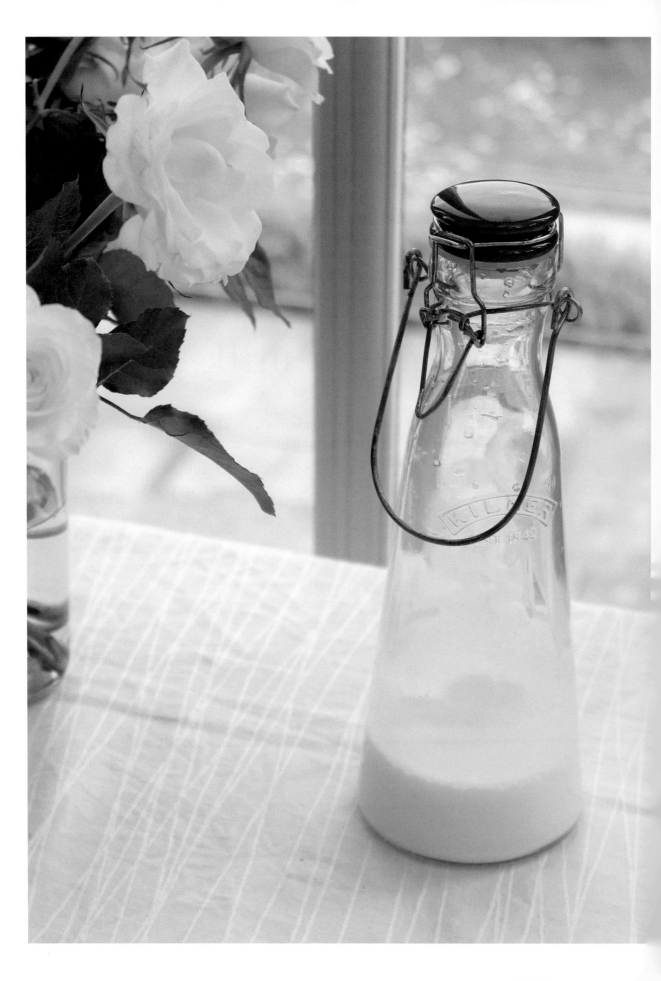

Cashew milk

1 cup raw, organic cashews
2 cups of filtered water

In a bowl, cover the cashews with filtered water and make sure there is enough water for them to expand.

Leave to soak overnight, or for a minimum of four hours.

Drain, rinse and put the cashews into a blender together with the fresh, filtered water and blend until smooth and creamy.

Cashew milk is really lovely when left unstrained, as it becomes thick and creamy and tastes super delicious. You can, however, strain it through a muslin cloth or nut bag for a thinner consistency if you wish. The creamier milk can be helpful if you are looking to put on more weight, which I was after the Paddison Program elimination diet once I was able to have nuts again. As always, I would have it with fresh leafy greens on the side to help break it all down.

Pour the milk over your porridge or use in other recipes. Keep refrigerated in a glass bottle - it lasts about three days.

Oat milk

I love oat milk and use it a lot in my cooking, since I was able to start having it earlier than I could anything made with nuts. It is especially good in hot cacao drinks and porridge.

$^1/_{10}$ rolled oats to
$^9/_{10}$ filtered water

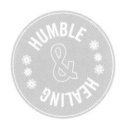

Blend until you have a milk-like consistency.

Pour into a glass bottle.

Alternatively, you can strain the oat milk through a nut milk bag or a muslin bag into a glass bottle using a funnel.

It keeps in the fridge for a few days; just shake it before you use it or blend it again.

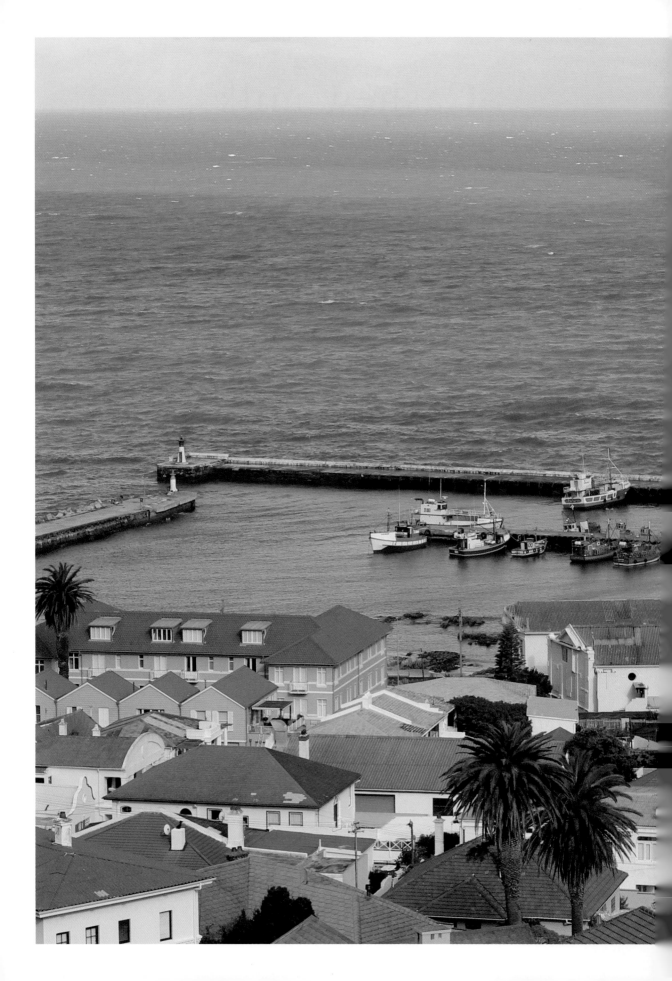

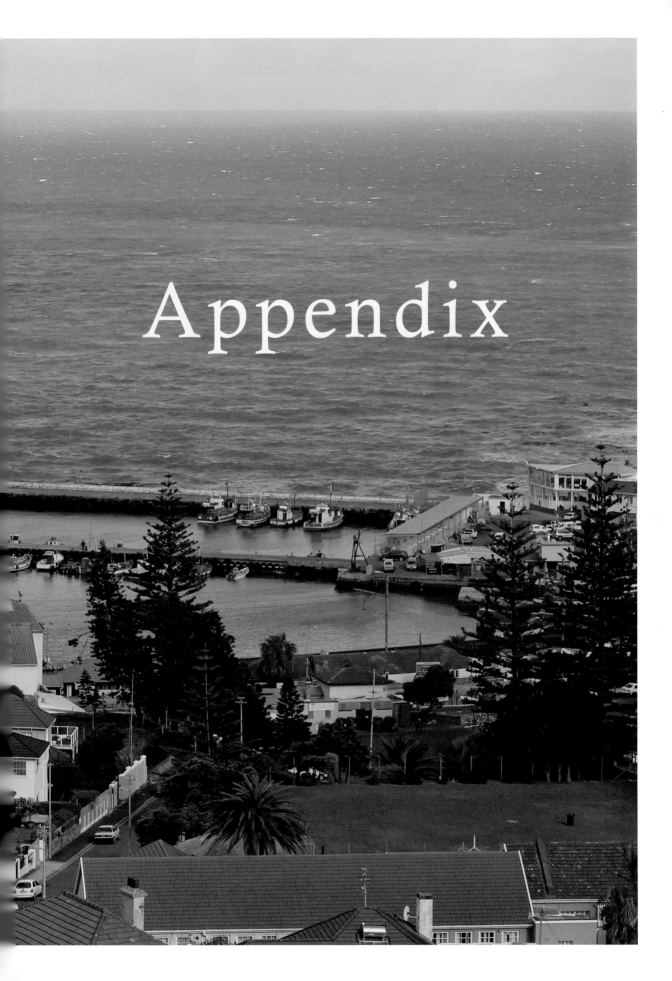

Appendix

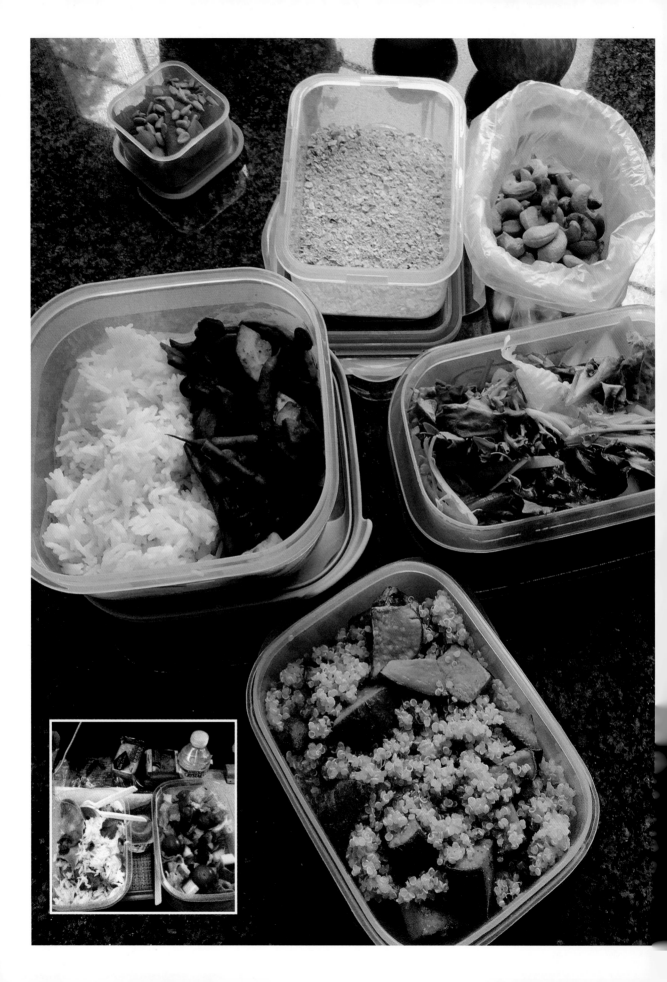

Travelling

—✦✦✦—

How do you travel when on a specific diet? Will you have to call the airline ahead of time to order a special meal? How about if you are travelling to a wedding – what do you tell the bride and the groom? And how about organising your food while in a new city? By now I have been there, done that numerous times and can share my best advice with you.

Instead of calling the airline to ask for a specific meal, just bring your own. You don't want to risk getting stuck with a 'vegan option' consisting of only a few salad leaves on a trans-Atlantic flight. On a long haul flight I often follow a recipe from the Paddison Program called Mega miso soup, which means that I pack a big container of Basmati rice with a dollop of brown rice miso paste, and some seaweed crumbled on top. I then bring a separate container with a huge, yummy salad. Once on the plane I just ask for a mug of hot water, which I use to blend the miso paste with the rice to create a miso soup and then enjoy this most delightful meal. As a snack I bring some fruit, buckwheat pancakes (page 45) or sushi rolls (page 64).

When flying to New York from London I had my leftover rice and salad for breakfast, which the stewardess had very kindly put in a fridge overnight. Spicy sweet potato wedges in a quinoa salad is also a safe bet as it keeps you full for a long time, is easy to pack and is super-delicious. For breakfast I just bring a container with some oats, cinnamon and dried fruits and nuts, and ask for some hot water in the morning to make porridge.

It is always great to see a Prêt a Manger at the airport, as they have many smoothies that are great to bring on a flight. They also have some lovely coconut water, which I have found to be perfect for keeping hydrated on the flight.

I always drink lots of water and tend to do a lot of yoga stretches on any flight to stop my joints from getting stiff. Before I had learned to bring down the inflammation in my joints with the Paddison Program, this was especially important to avoid an unpleasant awakening the next morning. These days I no longer suffer from any stiffness or extra pain after a flight but I still like to move around a fair bit during the longer flights.

For the flight back from your holiday you might not have the chance to cook your own food, so just pop into a restaurant and ask for some steamed rice and a big salad on the day of your return. I find that rice keeps me really full and energised and most restaurants will have it on the menu, but you can obviously choose anything that can be eaten cold – quinoa salads are perfect as well.

Left: Food for a 12 hour flight, which ended up being 16 hours including the time spent at the airports and travel time to and from the airports. Inset photo: My own food brought in Tupperware. I can then pick and choose the bits that work for me from what is being served – usually the bottled water and a plain salad. The crackers etc. need to find another home.

In another city

If you are on a very strict diet you might want to invest in a super-cute travel rice cooker, so that you know for sure that you will always have some backup food in your hotel room.

Staying in an apartment hotel rather than a hotel might also be a good idea, as having your own kitchen makes life much easier.

I had just started the Paddison Program when I went to New York for a friend's wedding and I stuffed my mini fridge to the brim with the most wonderful plant-based foods. I also learnt the locations of all the Whole Foods stores in NYC – that place is just the best when you are going plant-based. There are also some useful apps available (try HappyCow) for finding vegan restaurants.

Most hotels will have porridge on their breakfast menu, so just make sure it has been made with only oats, water and salt, then add fruit and nuts from the breakfast buffet, and maybe some bread if you are sure that there is no nasty stuff in it. You can even have a green salad on the side. The salad-part might sound crazy to you right now, but once you have been on a plant-based diet for a few months it makes complete sense. You start rethinking your old habits and listening to your body in a whole new way, and everything just tastes so good that you don't really care at what time of the day you are having porridge or a salad. Also, always pack a couple of spare Tupperware containers and some glass jars for transporting your food around on your holiday. As for going to restaurants, it can be helpful to contact them ahead of your visit, so that they can make preparations if necessary (yes, a lot of places will do that). Almost all restaurants that I have been to have been super-accommodating but the occasional one has not wanted to help out, and in those cases I have just left and gone elsewhere and always found another great place with delicious food, so no big deal!

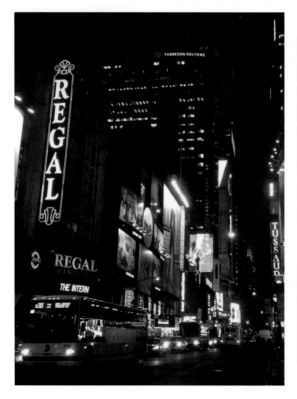

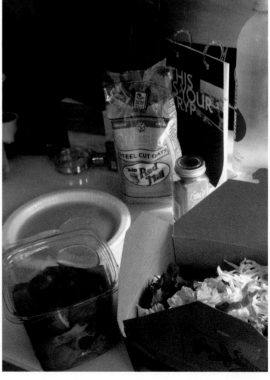

Shopping list

With the cupboards and fridge stocked with beautiful wholefoods, it is easy to prepare delicious meals quickly at all times. Choose organic and local where you can – farmers' markets are the best as you can buy lots of fruits and vegetables for less money. There is no need to have all the ingredients at home all the time, just keep rotating them for interesting and nutritious meals.

Vegetables, fruits and berries

Apples	Courgettes	Lettuce	Shallots
Aubergines	Garlic	Mangoes	Spinach
Bananas	Ginger, fresh	Onions – red and	Squash
Blueberries	Grapes	yellow	Strawberries
Bok choi	Green peas, frozen	Oranges	Sweet potatoes
Broccoli	Herbs, fresh – basil,	Papaya	Swiss chard
Carrots	dill, oregano,	Pears	Tomatoes
Cauliflower	rosemary, etc	Pineapple	Turmeric, fresh
Chillies, fresh	Kale	Potatoes	
Collard greens	Lemon	Raspberries	

Bread

Gluten in spelt is easier to digest so that has worked well for me. Finnish rye bread has been another good option. I look forward to eventually including wholewheat bread and also pasta in my diet, but for now I am keeping wheat to a minimum, so these are what I would recommend:

Sourdough spelt bread
Quinoa and amaranth bread
Finnish sourdough rye bread made without yeast

Fermented foods

Fermented foods contain good bacteria in the shape of probiotics that improve digestion and boost immunity. It is great to see more and more being written about how a healthy balance in the gut affects our physical, mental and emotional wellbeing; it is a good idea therefore always to have some fermented foods in the house. Choose unpasteurised versions as the probiotic bacteria are killed off in the pasteurisation process, which defeats our purpose. Some good options to try are:

Apple cider vinegar
Brown rice miso paste
Kimchi
Sauerkraut

Grains, pasta and noodles

Basmati rice – However, note that I found white rice to be slightly less acidifying than brown rice, so while my gut was healing, white Basmati rice was a good option. Once you can tolerate brown rice you have a wonderfully nutritious grain in your diet.

Arborio (risotto) rice
Porridge rice
Wild rice

Brown rice pasta (elbow macaroni, fusilli, penne, spaghetti) – I love my pasta, so cutting out wheat was quite traumatic… for about a minute until I discovered brown rice pasta. The consistency is so similar to regular pasta that I was happy; this is very important as obviously no one is interested in mushy pasta.

Corn pasta
Spelt lasagne sheets

Buckwheat grouts
Quinoa
Gluten-free oats
Gluten-free jumbo oats
Steel-cut oats – also known as 'Pinhead oats'

Rice noodles
Rice vermicelli noodles – white and brown
Rice paper – for making Summer rolls (page 80)

Nuts and seeds

Raw almonds
Raw cashew nuts
Raw walnuts
Pine nuts

Sunflower seeds
Pumpkin seeds

Beans and lentils

Dried or canned, where the canned options are good for making a meal quickly:
Adzuki beans
Black beans
Butter beans
Cannellini beans
Chickpeas
Lentils (red, black, green etc)

Spices and seasoning

Some of the recipes may seem to have rather a long list of ingredients, but it is usually because they contain a delicious mix of spices. By having all the following spices at home you will be able easily to make all the recipes in this book:

Black pepper
Cayenne pepper
Cinnamon – Ceylon cinnamon, sticks and powdered
Chilli flakes and powder
Cumin, ground
Curry powder - that contains only spices and herbs and no preservatives or bulking agents – always check the ingredients!
Ginger, dried
Organic herb salt – my favourite is A. Vogel's Herbamare, which is found in most health food shops and also at many of the regular grocery stores

Herbes de Provence
Himalayan pink salt
Maple syrup
Nutmeg - ground or whole for grating
Oregano - dried
Tamari sauce
Turmeric - powdered

References

1. Campbell TC, Campbell TM. *The China Study* First BenBella Books, Paperback Edition 2006 p. 12-20

2. Pulde A, Lederman M. *The Forks Over Knives Plan*. Simon & Schuster 2014 pp. 4-5, 16-17

3. Campbell TC, Campbell TM. *The China Study*. First BenBella Books, Paperback Edition 2006 p.31

4. McDougall J. When Friends Ask: Where Do You Get Your Protein? *The Dr McDougall Newsletter* April 2007 Vol. 6, No. 4. Page 2. www.drmcdougall.com/misc/2007nl/apr/dairy.pdf (accessed 15 May 2018)

5. Pulde A, Lederman M. *The Forks Over Knives Plan*. Simon & Schuster 2014, page 69

6. Mangels R. Protein in the vegan diet. In: Wasserman D, Mangels R. *Simply Vegan* 5th Edition, 2013: Vegetarian Resource Group. www.vrg.org/nutrition/protein.php (accessed 15 May 2018)

7. McDougall J. When Friends Ask: Where Do You Get Your Calcium? *The Dr McDougall Newsletter* February 2007 Vol. 6, No. 2. Page 1. www.drmcdougall.com/misc/2007nl/feb/calcium.pdf (accessed 15 May 2018)

8. Campbell TC, Campbell TM. *The China Study* First BenBella Books, Paperback Edition 2006 p. 205[9]

9. Mangels R. Iron in the Vegan Diet. In: *Simply Vegan* 5th Edition. (referring to Hallberg L. Bioavailability of dietary iron in man. *Ann Rev Nutr* 1981;1:123-147. DOI: 10.1146/annurev.nu.01.070181.001011)

www.vrg.org/nutrition/iron.php#r4 (accessed 15 May 2018)

10. Pulde A, Lederman M. *The Forks Over Knives Plan*. Simon & Schuster 2014, page 38

11. Campbell TC, Campbell TM. *The China Study*. First BenBella Books, Paperback Edition 2006 p. 232

12. McDougall J. When Friends Ask: Why Do You Avoid Adding Vegetable Oils? *The Dr McDougall Newsletter* August 2007 Vol. 6, No. 8. Page 1. www.drmcdougall.com/misc/2007nl/aug/oils.htm (accessed 15 May 2018)

13. Devkota S, Wang Y, Musch MW, Leone V et al. Dietary-fat-induced taurocholic acid promotes pathobiont expansion and colitis in Il10-/- mice. *Nature* 2012; 487(7405): 104–108. DOI:10.1038/nature11225

14. Mielants H, De Keyser F, Baeten D, Van den Bosch F. Gut inflammation in the spondyloarthropathies. *Current Rheumatology Reports* 2005; 7(3): 188–194.

15. Klaper M. Olive Oil is Not Healthy. Dr Klaper's talk at the Healthy Lifestyle Expo 2012 https://doctorklaper.com/videos/olive-oil-not-healthy/ (accessed 15 May 2018)

16. Esselstyn CB. Why does the diet eliminate oil entirely? *Dr. Esselstyn's Prevent & Reverse Heart Disease Program* www.dresselstyn.com/site/why-does-the-diet-eliminate-oil-entirely/ (accessed 15 May 2018)

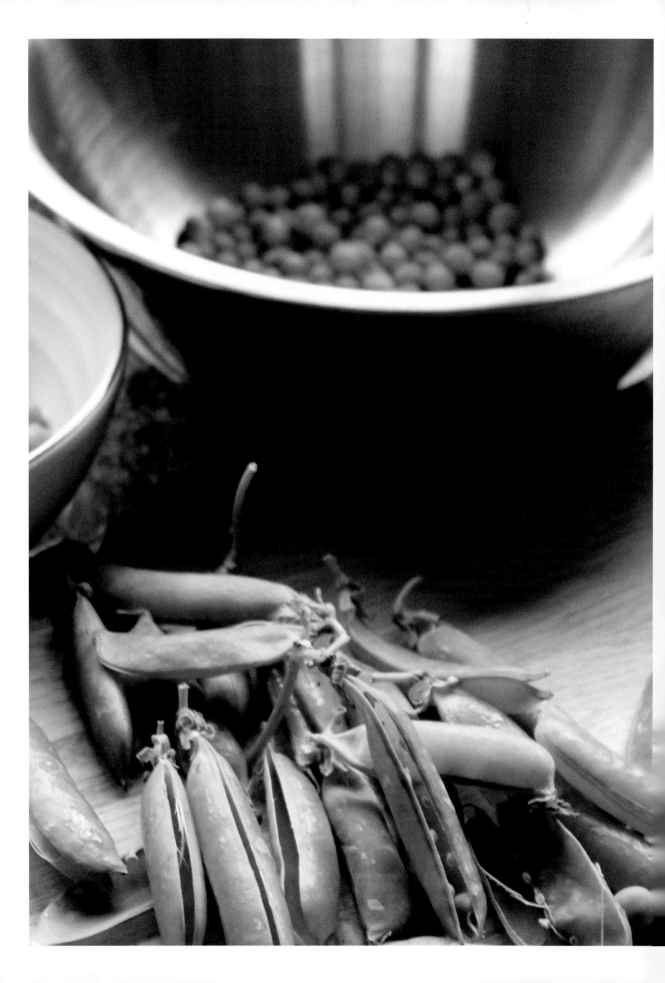

Index